Still
Beautiful

KATIE PIPER

Still Beautiful

**On Age, Beauty &
Owning Your Space**

Penguin Random House
DK [RED]

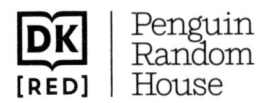

First published in Great Britain in 2025 by
DK RED, an imprint of
Dorling Kindersley Limited
20 Vauxhall Bridge Road,
London SW1V 2SA

The authorised representative in the EEA is
Dorling Kindersley Verlag GmbH. Arnulfstr. 124,
80636 Munich, Germany

Copyright © 2025 Dorling Kindersley Limited
A Penguin Random House Company
10 9 8 7 6 5 4 3 2
002–345496–Jun/2025

Text copyright © 2025 Katie Piper

Katie Piper has asserted her right to
be identified as the author of this work.

All rights reserved.
Cover photography: Sophia Spring

No part of this publication may be reproduced, stored in or introduced into a retrieval system, or transmitted, in any form, or by any means (electronic, mechanical, photocopying, recording, or otherwise), without the prior written permission of the copyright owner. The views and opinions expressed in this book are those of the author and do not necessarily reflect the views or positions of the publisher.
DK values and supports copyright. Thank you for respecting intellectual property laws by not reproducing, scanning or distributing any part of this publication by any means without permission. By purchasing an authorised edition, you are supporting writers and artists and enabling DK to continue to publish books that inform and inspire readers.
No part of this publication may be used or reproduced in any manner for the purpose of training artificial intelligence technologies or systems. In accordance with Article 4(3) of the DSM Directive 2019/790, DK expressly reserves this work from the text and data mining exception.

A CIP catalogue record for this book
is available from the British Library.
TPB ISBN: 978-0-2417-9428-9

Printed and bound in the United Kingdom

www.dk.com

MIX
Paper | Supporting responsible forestry
FSC™ C018179

This book was made with Forest Stewardship Council™ certified paper – one small step in DK's commitment to a sustainable future. Learn more at **www.dk.com/uk/information/sustainability**

To all those who have empowered me – there are so many of you! I try to pay it back by paying it forward

And to each person reading this book – may it help you to find healing and discover the untapped power within

'Everybody should read this book. The reflections into how Katie has shown resilience in the face of adversity are truly universal.'
Shirley Ballas, dancer & presenter

'A beautifully thoughtful, considered and candid read. As always, Katie's trademark warmth and grace shines through. Her tendency to lean into the joy means I can't WAIT TO hit 40! Another TRIUMPH Piper!'
Stacey Dooley, presenter & author

'This book has reframed my whole understanding of ageing. Katie's remarkable story has captured my heart for a long time - and this is her next chapter.'
Christine Lampard, presenter & broadcaster

'*Still Beautiful* invites us to reimagine what ageing and beauty should look like. Through Katie's powerful story, she teaches us that beauty is not in the eye of the beholder, but an intrinsic superpower that we define by just being (ourselves).'
Dame Denise Lewis,
Olympic champion, presenter & author

'Katie is one of the most important voices today. She is motivating without being preachy. When Katie writes it's from the heart and her heart is full of love. She is always willing to help anyone and everyone and through her writing, she does exactly that!'
Gaby Roslin, presenter & broadcaster

'I want to buy this book for every woman in my life! Katie encourages the reader to self-reflect and to learn about and embrace who they truly are where it matters... on the inside. She speaks from a place of her own unique experiences but with a powerful voice which will resonate with everyone who reads this book.'
Lauren Silverman,
Patron of the Katie Piper Foundation

'A distinctive, rare gem of a book packed with raw, unfiltered honesty. I found myself both nodding along and feeling lightbulbs go on. I want to be in Katie's tribe and you will too.'
Ranvir Singh, journalist & presenter

'Raw, brave and beautifully written. This is a book we all need to guide us into our second chapter with grace, resilience, appreciation and a sense of self-worth.'
Lisa Snowdon, presenter & model

'Katie has written this book so that we are in her story with her but she wants us to think about the lessons we can all learn as they are universal. More power to you, Katie Piper, you're wonderful.'
Carol Vorderman, broadcaster & author

Contents

Introduction   11

1. Age v. maturity   18
2. What am I worth?   34
3. Saying goodbye to the old you   56
4. Own your story   76
5. Finding purpose   98
6. Happily ever after?   120
7. Old is not a dirty word   148
8. A change of perspective   170
9. Take up the space   184
10. Life is hard, but you are resilient   208
11. Making peace with death   232

Epilogue   248
Acknowledgements   254
Notes   256

Introduction

When I turned 24, I felt invincible. Petite, pretty, blonde, I was bursting with energy and doing everything I could to make it as a model and presenter.

I'd been signed by a model agency and worked hard to stay slim so I could keep getting booked for shoots wearing tiny bikinis for the lads' mags that were so popular at the time. There had been some TV work, too, mostly presenting on shopping channels or hosting quiz shows on satellite channels, but I knew this was just the beginning. I was determined to do everything I could to 'make it', to go as far as possible. As my background was in beauty therapy, I knew how to make the most of my assets. The flat chest that had made me self-conscious as a teenager was taken care of with a credit card and an operation, boosting my confidence. I was too young to question the narrative I'd been fed and I traded on my looks, living recklessly and unaware of my own mortality. I smoked, I drank, and I didn't think about my diet beyond what would keep me slim. Words like 'ageing' and 'disability' had no place in my world.

At this point, I'd left behind the small town where I'd grown up and was living in a rented flat in north London with a group of friends. It was sparsely furnished, but we were incredibly house-proud. I loved the independence it represented, even if it did leave my bank account depleted at the end of each month.

I was too young to question the narrative I'd been fed and I traded on my looks, living recklessly and unaware of my own mortality.

Three or four nights a week, my flatmates and I would spend hours getting ready over multiple bottles of wine, then head out to the exclusive clubs (our modelling agency put us on the clubs' guest lists). Inside, rich men paid for the tables and endless bottles of champagne, hoping to impress the prettiest girls.

When I was in a relationship and spent the night with a boyfriend, I would wake up early and sneak into the bathroom, so I could brush my teeth, wash my face, and quickly put on a bit of make-up and perfume, then head back to bed and pretend to be asleep. Women on the TV programmes I watched always woke up looking beautiful, so I thought it was expected that I should look good at all times too. Back then, I worried about the smallest things. I had no way of knowing that my life was soon going to change for ever.

A few months later, outside my flat and in broad daylight, the act of one man flinging acid at me left me fighting for my life and needing to be put into an induced coma. Even once I was out of the coma, there was a long sequence of hundreds of operations and I had a lifetime of rehabilitation ahead of me. Those few seconds outside my flat that day split my life into before and after. My youth and my beauty – the two things I'd built my life around – were gone. I had also come close to death (not for the last time, but more on that later).

When I turned 40, people started asking me how I felt about this milestone. The clear implication was that I would feel sad or even horrified, but my honest answer was, 'I am *thrilled*.' I couldn't believe how blessed I was to be heading into a fifth decade. What a gift!

All this got me thinking – about life, death, youth, beauty, the way society tells us how we should look and behave as we get older, the ageism we see all around us and have internalised without question. And that's when the idea for this book began to form.

Ageing is a privilege that is denied to many. My life could have been over at 24. Gone, just like that. But, instead, I'm here, and I get to live another day, riding out the highs and lows of each passing year. So I wrote this book to challenge us to think about what we've been told, about our life being over once we reach a certain age, and society's obsession with beauty and youth.

The acid attack meant I had to learn, in the most brutal way possible, that I am more than what I look like on the surface. But we are *all* so much more than our age or our looks – that's what excites me. The power we have when we refuse to be sidelined just because we've passed a milestone birthday; the peace we find when we stop pretending that we're not ageing and accept it in all its glory; the joy we feel when we let go of what society thinks about us and finally live how we want to live.

But let me be honest from the start. I'm not saying that I have all the answers – I just want to open up a conversation about what we've consumed from the culture around us and how it forms what we feel about ourselves and our futures, so we can decide what's true. I want to empower us to reimagine ageing. What if it's not all doom and gloom like we've been told? What if, instead of only looking at the things it can take from us, we looked at what we gain as we get older, like wisdom, purpose, passion, and power? What if ageing is the magic key to letting go of other people's expectations and truly starting to live how we want to live? That sounds like something to celebrate to me.

Ageing is a privilege that is denied to many.

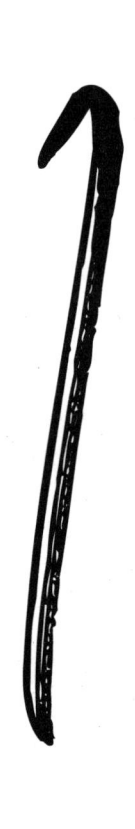

Age v. maturity

I was fortunate enough to have a safe and innocent childhood, growing up in a small, rural town alongside my older brother and younger sister. Our dad was the local barber and our mum a teacher in a nearby school. The biggest issue for me was that I wanted more than our sleepy little town could offer. I was hungry for the excitement and experiences of a big city – and my independence – so I moved out at the age of 17. First, I lived locally, studying to be a beautician at college while working at a supermarket in the evenings and at weekends to earn some cash, so I could move to London. I thought I was grown up, in the way that independent young people do. I had no idea how young and innocent I really was and that I would soon find myself having to mature overnight.

Some of you will know a bit of my story – how an acid attack orchestrated by a man I had briefly been seeing changed everything and catapulted me into ageing dramatically. In those torturous first moments when it happened, the sulphuric acid began to eat away at my skin, burning me and causing indescribable agony. It didn't seem humanly possible to survive that much pain. As the acid dripped down my face and into my eyes, I began to stumble around, unable to see but desperate to find help as the acid destroyed whatever it came into contact with. The pain began to overwhelm me and I thought I was about to die. Part of me welcomed the idea – anything to escape the agony I was in. I drifted in and out of consciousness and woke up in hospital, so disorientated that I was unsure whether I was dead or alive.

Within days, I had the first of many operations. This one was to remove the dead skin and begin to rebuild my face. After another op shortly after, I had to be put into an induced coma for 12 days because the resulting pain would have been too difficult to bear if I'd been conscious. I'd suffered third-degree burns, meaning all three layers of my skin had been destroyed. I'd lost most of my nose, my eyelids, and half my left ear. My eyes, mouth, and tongue were all damaged, my neck and cleavage badly burned, and splashes of acid had caused damage to the skin on my hands, arms, and legs. It wasn't just the features of my face that had been affected but my entire face had been eroded in places.

I woke from the coma to a life that was unrecognisable. I was fully dependent on other people – doctors, nurses, my family, and friends – for everything. My former independent life as an able-bodied 24-year-old woman was gone. Whereas before I would happily wolf down a takeaway, now I had to be fed through a drip into my stomach because the acid had damaged my oesophagus so badly. I had taken for granted being able to go to the toilet whenever I needed to, but now I couldn't get up to use the bathroom so was dependent on a catheter. My previously good eyesight was badly damaged, leaving me vulnerable and able to do very little unaided. When I was able to get out of bed, many weeks later, I had to use a wheelchair as I was too weak to walk. My muscles were wasting from lack of use, and I was losing weight and strength, unable to build myself up with food and exercise. So many basic bodily functions that I hadn't even thought twice about just before the attack were now impossible for me. My independence, my youth, didn't feel like it was fading away, it was gone – just like that.

The damage wasn't only physical, of course. I was deeply traumatised by the acid attack, but the man who arranged it had also raped me in a hotel room just days before. He was so violent that I'd barely escaped from the hotel with my life. That alone had been enough to turn my life upside down and leave me shell-shocked and petrified, but then to find that he'd arranged for another man to viciously assault me with acid? I had no way of processing everything that had happened. I had no frame of reference for such acts of violence, things I would never have imagined happening to me, nor to anyone I knew. I was terrified and didn't feel safe anywhere, even in the hospital. Both my attackers were walking free and I was convinced they would come back to finish me off. I was in fear of my life 24/7, dreaming feverishly that I wasn't even safe in the hands of the doctors and nurses who were doing their best to help me.

When I was released from hospital, I wasn't able to return to my flat, so I went back home to live with my parents. I was dependent on them for the physical and emotional support I needed to get me through each day. Unsurprisingly, given all I was going through, I found that I couldn't relate to people my age any more. I felt decades older than I had just months previously. Conversations then had been about where to go out drinking, what to wear, or what the latest modelling opportunity was. But now, suddenly, my life was all about my medical needs. My friends were worried about whether replying straight away to a text from someone they fancied was too keen; I was concerned about whether I'd ever be able to eat solid food again. It wasn't that I begrudged them the position they were in – I was glad

Maturity isn't about age: it's about experience and mindset.

they weren't living through the hell I was – but I just couldn't relate to their lives in the same way any more.

The attack forced me to grow up in the most brutal way. Yes, it aged me physically – by inflicting more damage to my body than most people deal with in their entire lives – but also I had to grow up emotionally. I look back now and think that there was a naivety to the way I lived up until that point, as though nothing could ever hurt me. My safe upbringing and experiences meant I'd been sheltered from some of life's cruelties.

Going through such trauma made me realise that maturity isn't about age; it's about experiences and mindset. Many people have to confront difficult situations well before I did, and when these happen in childhood or adolescence, the maturing process is speeded up. Losing a parent or sibling, living in an abusive home environment, having caring responsibilities for someone else in our household – all these kinds of challenges force those going through them to find ways to cope that the average child doesn't have to.

One of my first boyfriends had grown up in the care system and then lived in a rented bedroom in a house. He was always working, turning his hand to all sorts of jobs so he could pay his bills, as there were no parents at home he could call on if he was ever a bit short. Hanging out in his room one day, I noticed that he had tinned meat, tuna, and sardines lined up in his wardrobe. 'Why have you got all this army food?' I asked him, confused. 'If I leave it in the kitchen it gets nicked,' he explained, 'and I can't afford to get any more, so I buy what I need for the month when I get paid and I keep it all in here.' It was an eye-opener for me – a world away from my comfortable home life where the cupboards and fridge were magically restocked without me having to do anything. The money I earned at that time from part-time jobs was for clothes, magazines, and going out; I didn't have to budget to make sure I had the basics to keep me alive.

I look back now and can see that he experienced a similar isolation from his peers that I did after the attack. I could rebel against my parents when I was a teenager, secure in the knowledge that they loved me and would be there for me no matter what, but he had needed to become fiercely independent and had no one to fall back on. The things I took for granted at home – the hugs, kind words, even the stupid arguments that got quickly forgotten – he had only ever dreamed of. Whether you're in care, a teenage mum, a young carer, or have suffered a life-changing injury, you find yourself in a place where your concerns are not those of the average person your age. Your experiences don't match up with theirs. The thoughts that consume your mind and the activities filling your day may vary hugely from theirs.

It's easy to pity people in these situations and, as someone who's been on the receiving end of that, I get it. No one would wish pain or suffering on anyone – especially a child or young person. But I think that by only seeing people who've been through hard experiences as the object of pity, we often miss something key: they have usually learned a lot. They've often gained a level of maturity and wisdom that people years older than them have yet to do. They've faced some of the hardest situations that life can throw at you and they've kept going. Wisdom, resilience, and maturity don't land in your lap at a certain age, like a birthday gift from the universe. They can only be gained by means of experience.

We sometimes say things like, 'Oh, I would never have been able to handle that', but the truth is, we don't know what we can handle until we're in the middle of it. It's in life's testing moments that we

Wisdom, resilience, and maturity don't land in your lap at a certain age, like a birthday gift from the universe. They can only be gained by means of experience.

discover there's a steely determination in us to keep going. If we let them, the experiences we have – the good, the bad, and the ugly – can help inform how we tackle a similar situation in the future. We build confidence in ourselves and the ability to handle the tough stuff. I often say that, after what I've been through, there's nothing that could flatten me. I will still have bad days or times when things feel overwhelming, but I've learned from dealing with much worse, day in and day out, that I can do it. In many ways, it's like maturity is gradually built from the data of doing the everyday, but those tough times, ones that call for us to step up, increase this data acquisition process tenfold. There are young carers who, at the age of eight, in many ways, are far more mature than some 25-year-olds who still live at home and have a parent who does their washing. Because, despite being so young, there is no one else there to do the food shopping, make the meals, clean the house, or provide emotional support to parents or siblings, so they have had to learn what to do and get on with it.

One of the biggest lessons I had to learn as I was recovering is that we can't choose what happens to us, but we can choose how we respond. Sometimes we wish we could turn back the clock and change things. I can't tell you the hours I spent thinking, 'What if I'd never met that man? What if I hadn't gone to meet him the weekend he attacked me? What if I hadn't left my flat the day of the acid attack?' There are a million 'What ifs' for all of us, but I realised that desperately longing for things to be different was getting me nowhere. The energy we spend doing this can be used to work out how to deal with the things that are. For me, I came to see that there was no point comparing my life to the lives of others my age and wishing I could return to who I was before the attack; things had changed irrevocably. I had to decide whether what happened to me would be the thing that would define me

Pain and trauma are inevitable but they don't have to be a life sentence.

and I would wither away and let it destroy me, or I would rebuild my life out of what had been taken. I'm not saying that happened overnight. We can't skip grief and pretend hard things aren't happening to us (this topic is so important, we'll return to it in Chapter 10), but I slowly came to realise that I needed to take what I'd been through and learn from it and grow.

I'm sure as you look back over your life, you'll find that it hasn't all been plain sailing. Maybe you experienced some trauma when you were young or something happened more recently, but there will have been times when things didn't go your way or events unfolded in a way that you never would have chosen for yourself or for your loved ones. I hope you can look back and give yourself some credit for keeping going, getting through it, and not letting it defeat you. Some days we might feel like we've done little more than exist but, importantly, we're still here. If we're putting one foot in front of the other – even if we're shuffling along – we're still moving forwards.

I hope that, from all these reflections, you can see what life's challenges have taught you, how they've made you who you are today. If it hadn't been for the attack, I would have carried on with a fairly superficial, self-serving life, more worried about how I looked than the best ways to have a positive impact on the world. I am the person I am today because of the adversities I've overcome.

So, while the surgeons rebuilt my face on the outside, I had to take care of the inside – no one else could do that for me. Maturing is inner work and it's a choice. The ageing process happens to us all: we are passive participants in it and can't do anything to stop the passage of time. No matter how many anti-ageing products we buy, we will continue to age until the day we die. However, maturing is optional. It's the work we can choose to do to look after our inner wellbeing, and each year offers us opportunities to grow and develop. It's taking what life throws our way and making the best of it, knowing that pain and trauma are inevitable but they don't have to be a life sentence. It's learning from every experience, whether it's good or bad.

I try to step back from each situation that I find hard or stressful and give myself some time to think before I react. As I've got older, I've realised that's one of the best ways to let my ego calm down, so I can choose how I *really* want to respond. Sometimes I need to get out and exercise to release some of the stress from my body and to give myself some headspace. I journal each day, writing notes on my phone that allow me to get all sorts of thoughts out of my head and on to the page instead. We're all made differently, so each of us has different processes that work for us, but a common one would be talking to someone to help process things we're finding hard. I have had therapy on and off over many years and it's been incredibly helpful in helping me to grow and move past the places where I would have become stuck if I'd tried to deal with them alone. For many, just talking to a partner or a friend is enough to gain a fresh perspective on what's troubling them.

We don't have to be thankful for everything we've been through to recognise that many of life's challenges also bring opportunities for us to grow. We can choose to look at each day and think, 'Did I learn something? Did I grow? Did I use the challenges before me as an opportunity to mature and to change?'

So, whatever life has thrown at you in the past, whatever comes your way today or tomorrow, my words of encouragement to you are that you don't let the hard things define you. We're all products of our past, but we don't have to be prisoners of it. Take the learnings, squeeze every last drop of wisdom out of them that you can, and know that the power to determine how you respond and who you become lies in one person: you. You can do this.

A moment to pause
•••

Getting older simply happens, but maturing is a choice. How can you reframe today's challenges as an opportunity for growth?

2

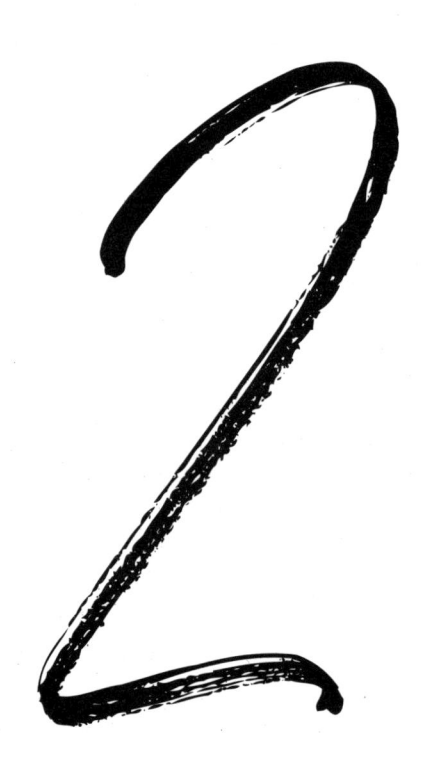

What am I worth?

Though acid attacks were quite rare in this country when it happened to me in 2008,[1] I always knew why my ex had chosen this form of violence. He wanted to take away what he thought was most important about me: my beauty. He believed that without my looks, I would be nothing, as I'd built my life around them. I'd certainly enjoyed 'pretty privilege' up to that point – by which I mean, men were attentive whether I was waiting to get served in a bar or needed a seat on the Tube. After my boob job, I got more attention straight away; it was crazy to see how much more noticeable I became when I went from being flat-chested to a C cup. Like many young women, I was yet to realise that founding my worth on what I looked like or what others (particularly men) thought about me was incredibly shaky ground.

There is so much that can be said about beauty and ageing. Many people try to retain their looks as they get older by following faddy diets and exercise patterns, buying the latest 'miracle' face creams, having plastic surgery, or getting expensive beauty treatments. There seems to be a strong association between youth and beauty when there is no basis for this. We've seen ever-younger women seeking out 'tweakments', a casual attitude to fillers among millennials and Gen Zs,[2] and people in their 20s and 30s getting 'prejuvenation Botox', to stop themselves

Our looks change throughout our lives, so they're a very unstable foundation on which to build our identity.

getting wrinkles.[3] But why? How much of this stems from being conditioned to see our looks as the basis of our worth?

In this chapter, we'll explore these and other aspects of beauty and ageing. The truth is that no diet or skin cream will truly help us to find our self-worth. Our looks change throughout our lives, so they're an unstable foundation on which to build our identity.

Of course, culture was and is obsessed with the way women look. As I was growing up, page after page of newspapers and magazines were devoted to what actresses and models wore, and every new haircut seemed worthy of appearing on their front pages. Each tiny perceived flaw was analysed and there was great speculation about weight lost or gained.

I was a huge fan of the Spice Girls and their 'Girl Power' message. I can still remember them bursting on to our TV screens in the music video for 'Wannabe', wearing what they wanted, dancing how they wanted, and being loud and proud. I watched them be assertive and unapologetic in interviews and it had a big impact on me, as young girl working out my own place in the world. But, despite their ethos of female empowerment they, too, were continually subjected to comments about their looks and weight. Victoria Beckham (aka Posh Spice) was not only asked about her post-pregnancy weight on national TV but also asked to get on a set of scales to prove her answer.[4] The front page of a national newspaper showed a picture of her the first time she left home after becoming a mum, with arrows pointing to each part of her body where they deemed she needed to lose weight.[5] It's hideous to think about what they went through now, but it was part and parcel of how women were treated at the time. Everything was up for grabs: cellulite, spots, rolls of flesh, sweat patches, birthmarks… all were criticised and critiqued as though they were of national importance.

For large numbers of women, this is the culture we've grown up in – being bombarded with this kind of thing during some of our most formative years. Thankfully, some things have changed since then, but the way women are viewed is still nowhere near on a par with how men are treated. It doesn't matter how accomplished women are – how intelligent, talented, and hard-working, or whether they've racked up Oscars and Grammys, worked on the highest-grossing films, or sold out huge stadiums – their physical appearance still comes under intense scrutiny. Actor Nicola Coughlan was told she was 'brave' for undertaking her role in the TV series *Bridgerton*, which involved a number of sex scenes. The not-so-subtle implication of this comment was that she was daring to show her body despite not conforming to the stereotype for the kind of character she was playing. Her comeback was spot on, that 'it is hard because I think women with my body type – women with perfect breasts – we don't get to see ourselves on screen enough'.[6]

Jameela Jamil, an actor who is also known for her @i_weigh Instagram account, once posted about the types of images the media has shared of her over the years.[7] She showed shots of herself at two different weights side by side and said that at the time when she was incredibly thin, she was hungry and unhappy, but when she was curvier, she was feeling successful and was very happy in her relationships. She says that the press consistently used shots of her smiling when she was thin and looking unhappier when she was heavier, cropping out friends who were with her to make it look like she was alone. The takeaway for the reader: thin equals happy and successful, curvy equals sad and unwanted.

It's not just in the entertainment business that this happens. When Theresa May was the UK's prime minister and Nicola

Sturgeon Scotland's first minister, there was an article on the front page of the *Daily Mail* that focused not on their policies but on their legs. Their legs! The two most senior political figures in the UK, meeting to talk about a Scottish referendum and Brexit – two of the most important political issues in their countries at the time – and a mainstream publication thought this was the time to pit them against one another in terms of their looks, saying that Nicola Sturgeon's legs were much more 'flirty' and 'tantalising' than Theresa May's.[8] When the *Daily Mail* was criticised for being so misogynistic, its response to people who were angry was for them to 'get a life' and it was just a 'light-hearted' piece.[9] In this are echoes of all the previous decades when women were pinched on the bum (or worse) by male bosses and then, if they complained, they were told that they couldn't take a joke. We see similar misogyny around the world, including comments and articles about Kamala Harris's clothing, while she was running for president of the USA, that we would be unlikely to see if the two candidates in the race were male.[10]

What does it tell us, and the women coming up behind us, when scrutiny of the appearance of female politicians far outweighs that of male ones? Some people say that women who work in the media are fair game for being criticised about their appearance. Whether you agree with that or not, surely men and women should be held to the same standards. Surely women entering whatever field of work they choose shouldn't find that the papers will be more interested in their legs than the words that come out of their mouth. These things should indeed be the case but, even in the business world, women say there is pressure on them to look polished, a pressure that just isn't on their male counterparts.[11] The bottom line is that women are still often reduced to what men think about their appearance. And it's in this landscape that we're trying to find our place in the world, our own sense of self-worth, and understand what we can bring to society.

I, too, was there. I was young, the time of life that is presented as the most beautiful, but my face was red raw and unrecognisable, covered by a clear plastic mask 23 hours a day. I had never seen anyone, of any age, look like I did. There was no diversity in the media at the time, and there was no Instagram for people with burns to be able to post pictures of themselves in the same way that anyone else might do. I didn't know who I was or how I would fit into the world.

When I ventured out of the safety of my parents' house some months after I left the hospital, I noticed that people didn't hold the door open for me. In fact, they often let it slam in my face. If I sat next to someone on the Tube, they would get up and move away, as though I had something contagious. In shops, when I needed to pay for something, people no longer smiled and said, 'Hello'; they struggled to meet my eyes and avoided small talk. It made me feel like the world had no use for me any more, as though I was invisible. That said, there were also times when I felt hyper-visible. People couldn't stop staring, never having seen anyone who looked like I did. It felt similar to being an animal in a cage – a curiosity to be judged by others. The amazing doctors and nurses treated me with such compassion and care, but the medical care system itself – being on a treadmill of appointments and protocols – often left me feeling like my identity was disabled and disfigured; a patient, not a person.

I felt desexualised too. Straight after the attack, some of the hair on my head had been burned, other bits had fallen out, and some was shaved off in the hospital, so my injuries and skin could be cleaned up and treated. Doctors and nurses would enter the room and have to ask whether I was male or female as it was impossible to tell from how I looked. My body had stopped feeling like my own. I couldn't perform basic functions for myself; I was reliant on others the whole time. Different nurses would bathe me, so I had no choice over who saw me naked. I lost all sense of dignity.

I'd always enjoyed my body and wasn't ashamed of it, so it wasn't that. It was more that I had enjoyed being a sexual being and having the power to present myself in the way I wanted to with clothes, make-up and shoes that fitted my mood. There was a sense of power and control about it, part of the statement I was making to the world about who I was.

In 2008, lads' mag culture had been rife for the best part of a decade. Publications such as *FHM, Nuts, Zoo,* and *Loaded* all carried pictures of women in bikinis (or less) on their front covers, and they were objectified by the writers and readers of the magazines. The criterion for who appeared in them? Women who were deemed hot. No one else was worth paying attention to. Our value came from the male gaze. Those who were considered worthy found it flattering, while those who weren't had a hard time criticising it without seeming sour. I was part of that industry for four years and, looking back, I see that, naively, I didn't realise how dark some parts of it were. The women involved were conditioned to underestimate themselves, to place their worth in their looks alone and not think about what else they had to contribute to society other than that.

As a model, I knew what it was like to be desired and to feel desirable. Now, I felt like a slab of meat – an object at the mercy of those who poked and prodded me. I couldn't even conceive of myself as sexy at that stage; I was simply trying to stay alive.

For others in the modelling world, this shift didn't come as fast or as dramatically as it had for me, but they still found that, as they aged, the work dried up and the attention they had been used to receiving moved away from them and on to the younger generation. It can be incredibly painful when your identity is based on your looks and you find that even as young as your late 20s, you're already considered to be 'past your best'. You can start to feel invisible and overlooked. The same is true of so many heterosexual women who, when they're dating, feel like men are looking for 'younger models' and so they feel invisible as they get older.

Getting into a relationship with a man wasn't on my own agenda at that point. After my brief but catastrophic interactions with the man who raped me and arranged the acid attack, it couldn't have been further from my mind. Like many rape survivors, I needed some time to recover physically and mentally before I could even think about being with a man. What I did have to think about, though, was what I was going to do for work.

At that time, no one wanted someone who looked like me to be in a magazine or on TV. I was disfigured, blind in one eye, and in and out of hospital for continual follow-up treatment and operations to allow me to breathe and eat. I was always fatigued, as your body burns twice as many calories when it's trying to heal. My hands were in splints to maintain mobility as the skin healed. I had never been academic and I'd known that from a young age, so instead I made the best of what I did have, but now that was gone. Even my fall-back career of beauty therapy wasn't an option – I couldn't see well enough to give people treatments and even if that wasn't the case, I found myself thinking, 'Who would want to be pampered by someone who looks like me?'

I was dealing with an extreme situation, but don't we all discount ourselves at different times? We think we're too short, too tall, too young, too old, too fat, too thin, our hair is too big or too flat, our shape too curvy or not curvy enough? We don't meet someone's definition of perfection and so we feel crap about ourselves. We see pictures in a magazine and think that we could never look like that, so we're not beautiful. But could any of us ever hope to emulate the smooth, blemish-free skin of the models who have spent hours in the chair of a make-up artist and, even after that, have had their images airbrushed? *No one looks like the models in magazines – not even the models themselves!* So who benefits from us judging ourselves by an impossible standard? Who benefits from us not feeling good enough? It's not us. We are pitted against one another, seeing whether we're prettier or sexier than the woman next to us so we can feel good about ourselves. The beauty industry in the UK alone was projected to be worth £12.93 billion (US$ 16.78 billion) in 2024, with estimates placing it at £1,178 billion ($1,436.7 billion) around the globe by 2027.[13] But 'beauty' is a made-up concept defined differently in different eras and by cultures around the world.

In the past 200 years, we've seen beauty standards come and go. There was the Victorian era, when the ideal look was being plump, having a full-figure but a cinched-in waist, which was followed by the androgynous look of the 1920s, when a flat chest was favoured. Fast forward to the golden age of Hollywood, from the 1930s to the 1950s, and curves were back in – the hourglass form of the famous Marilyn Monroe being the ideal – but, by the 1960s, everyone wanted to be thin and willowy with long, slim legs. In my lifetime, there's been the athletic build of the supermodels of the 1980s, the heroin chic of the 1990s, when

I had to dismantle the lie that my worth was in my looks and truly grasp the truth: there is more to each of us inside than what is on the outside.

models looked (and perhaps were) starved and, more recently, the Kim Kardashian look of large boobs and bum, but with a 'healthy-skinny' body, including a flat stomach and thigh gap.[14] Which of us can create curves when they are declared 'in' and then magically get them to disappear a few years later when a straighter silhouette is being touted as the ideal? Diets, surgery, and uncomfortable clothing choices (corsets anyone?) can only get us so far. The truth is that none of us can have a fashionable figure all our life – it's physically impossible.

That what is considered beautiful varies is clear from journalist Esther Honig's experiment. She sent a headshot of herself, with her hair pulled back and without make-up, to 25 Photoshop editors around the world, asking them to edit her face to reflect the beauty standards of their country.[15] The results are fascinating. Australia went for one of the most natural edits, focusing on adding tan and blusher, whereas Bangladesh gave her a luminous glow that even the best make-up in the world couldn't hope to recreate (imagine the aura of an angel). The Philippines gave her a smaller forehead, Greece crazy long eyelashes and India heavy eyebrows. In Pakistan, the editor considered she would be more beautiful with darker eyes, while Serbia wanted to highlight her blue eyes and make them bigger. The photo that came back from the USA was almost unrecognisable because of the changes made to her eye shape and hair.

As I said, beauty is a made-up construct, yet we're spending close to £13 billion a year in the UK alone trying to achieve it. Imagine what else could be done with that money. For years, the media has stoked our dissatisfaction with how we look and people have lined their pockets with money made from advertising revenues, diet products, and anti-ageing creams. But let's be clear: we will not find our self-worth by weighing less or trying to look younger. If we don't like who we are fundamentally, if we don't see that what's on the outside isn't the most important thing, we will spend our lives investing our time and energy in things that, ultimately, won't make us feel any better.

We've been conditioned to feel worthy when a man or woman looks our way approvingly. We are validated by feeling pretty and sexy and, equally, crushed when someone says something negative about our appearance. Have you ever thought about the double standards at play in all this? Why men walk around in shorts with hairy legs on full display, yet we would be horrified if we were caught with less than perfectly smooth skin? Why the majority of women wear make-up and so few men do? Why women are held to these impossible standards of perfection and men aren't? Why men get called 'silver foxes' by the media and 'distinguished' as they age, but there's no similar narrative for women with grey or white hair? Just to be clear, I'm not advocating for or against hairy legs, wearing make-up, or going grey. I'm just highlighting some of the hypocrisy about what is considered normal for men and for women and reminding you that, whatever you choose to do with your body, it has no impact on your worth.

One of the things I've consciously tried to do on social media is show the reality of what I look like. When I'm on TV, I've spent hours with people helping me to get ready, doing my hair and make-up, but it's not what I look like day to day. I decided that I would film or photograph myself wherever and whenever – whether I've just got out of bed, am sweaty from working out, or am in unflattering light – doing just normal, everyday things. I try not to edit or filter myself. It's not that I think I look great all the time – far from it – but it's one way I can make my life less about what I look like, and be real so people don't only ever see a polished version of me. Of course, the reality of social media is

At your funeral, no one will talk about your physical appearance, because that does not sum up who you are.

that when I'm not made up, plenty of people feel the need to comment and tell me how rough they think I look. Or to tell me I'm brave for showing myself as I really am. Those people are at least trying to be kind, but they don't realise how offensive they are being. Why is it brave to be myself? It can be hard not to take it personally, but I've developed a thick skin. When it comes to trolls, I try to remind myself it says more about them – that they would take time out of their day to insult someone on social media – than it does about me and my worth. It's also, surprisingly, made me more confident. When I meet people in person, I know they know what I actually look like and won't be expecting me to be ultra-glamorous.

The truth is, no one is 'beautiful' their entire lives or to everyone around them – especially if beauty is equated with youth. When we start to let go of the need to be physically beautiful, we realise that who we are is so much more important than what we look like. When I was recovering from the attack, I couldn't conceive that I would ever look in the mirror and be happy with what I saw. I had to start again and find a new way of relating to my body and understanding my place in the world. I had to dismantle the lie that my worth was in my looks and truly grasp the truth: there is more to each of us inside than what is on the outside.

Judging someone only on their looks is incredibly shallow. Most of us will have met people society would judge to be beautiful, but if they turn out to be rude or there doesn't seem to be much below the surface, their 'beauty' soon vanishes. We also will have experienced how truly beautiful someone becomes to us when we know them well and see the love and kindness they bring to those around them. The vast majority of us don't maintain relationships with people for years because of what they look like; we do so because of who they are. We often talk about people being attractive – again, meaning that they are physically appealing – but there are so many ways someone can be attractive. I don't know about you but I often find myself drawn to people on social media not because they have big eyes or a symmetrical face but because I find them interesting and inspiring. Being attractive is so much more than being good-looking!

It took me years to re-establish my sense of identity and to ground it in something more sustainable than my looks. I'll go on to share with you how finding a sense of purpose and realising what I could give to the world reshaped me and brought me to a better place. We'll explore how living our lives as our most authentic selves means letting go of some of this toxic obsession with our looks and finding out what our true value is.

For now, let me say that I've learned the importance of making peace with how I look. It is far more powerful than any treatment you'll find anywhere in the world. So much of that peace comes from not locating my self-worth in my outward appearance but from knowing that I am loved, valued, and valuable for so many other reasons. The more I discovered a sense of purpose in life and felt like I could contribute to society in different ways, the more at peace with myself I became and the less worried I was about how I looked. Discovering these things also helps as we age and our looks begin to change. If we put less emphasis on our body and more on everything else we have to offer, the less we will worry about our changing appearance. We can embrace our physical changes knowing that they don't define us and be aware that with each passing year we are growing into ourselves and increasing our awareness of who we are and what we bring to the world.

I'd lost so much because of the attack, but what I was fortunate to have was so much love from the people around me. My parents hadn't left my side since the accident. It didn't matter to them what I looked like – they loved me regardless, and they slept on a chair in my room if they had to, just to be near me. People I'd never met before, such as my doctors, nurses, and especially my incredible surgeon, Doctor Mohammad Ali Jawad, all poured out so much time and energy to help me when I was at my lowest. Dr Jawad pushed for pioneering treatments to be used on me, the first of their kind anywhere in the world. Why? I had nothing to offer. I wasn't famous, I couldn't afford to give him huge sums of money, and he knew very little about me or my life before the attack. He helped me because he saw me as deserving of care simply because I am a human being. With his charity work, Dr Jawad helps people around the world in positions similar to mine. He would have done it for anyone.

When you think about the people who know and love you, what do you think they love most about you? How plump your skin is? Your youth? The size of your thighs? Your latest hairstyle? I'd hazard a guess that those things wouldn't even make the top 20 in a list of what they'd say about you. I imagine they would focus on the fact that you make them laugh or you're quick to lend a hand or a listening ear when needed. If they commented on your smile, it wouldn't be because they cared whether your teeth were straight and brilliant white; it would be because they enjoy seeing you happy. At your funeral, no one will talk about your physical appearance, because that does not sum up who you are.

The world is obsessed with how we look, but what would happen if we chose to focus instead on who we are, our unique characteristics and qualities, our experiences and what we've overcome and achieved? I'm not saying that, if we did this we would have no more bad days when we feel rubbish about ourselves, but let's give ourselves the dignity of remembering that our worth is not wrapped up in our looks. How we appear on the outside is the least interesting thing about us. Your purpose here on this earth is not to win the approval of a fickle fashion and beauty industry or a random stranger on Instagram. You are worthy. Full stop.

A moment to pause
●●●

Which non-physical attribute do you love most about yourself? If your closest friends or family were to describe your best qualities, what would they say?

3

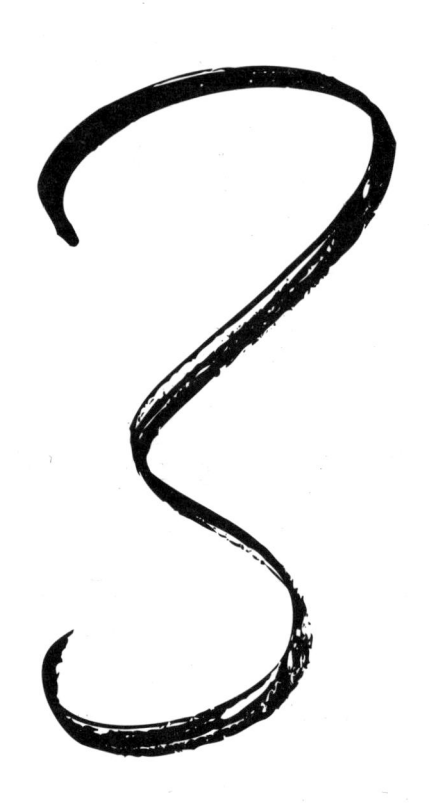

Saying goodbye to the old you

For years I would dream about my old face. I would see my wide smile, the cupid's bow of my lips, the flat, wide nose that I inherited from my mum's side of the family. I could remember what it felt like to wash my face and touch soft skin, to put on moisturiser and trace the contours of my cheekbones under my fingertips. In my dreams I was her once more, so when I woke up, I would be devastated all over again. Sometimes I would look at my old modelling shots and cry. I'd feel like an 80-year-old who shows someone photos of an unrecognisable version of themselves and says, 'I used to be a looker back in the day. I was quite pretty then you know.' It broke my heart that what was left of my face after the acid had melted away my features was removed and unceremoniously dumped in a medical waste bin. Although I was suddenly in a rare and extreme situation, I'm sure this feeling of longing to look how we used to look is entirely familiar to so many of us as one we have when we look in the mirror and see ourselves ageing.

When it comes to my own face and body, surgeons rebuilt me in the most incredible way – using cartilage from my rib to make my nose, and from my ears to create a new nostril – but I would never look like my old self physically again. I used to look like my mum and brother; now, I don't look like anyone in my family. I feared forgetting my old face, glad I enjoyed looking like I did

Youth is so idolised that we often have to grieve it before we can embrace the good things about our age.

while she was mine, but wishing I could take her out again one last time.

I remember trying on some of my old clothes and I couldn't imagine ever wearing them again. There were dresses I loved, but they no longer fitted with my lifestyle. It had changed so much that I was more comfortable in a hospital than I was in a nightclub. I'd lost so much weight that even my shoe size changed. I'd spent years and lots of money building my collection of heels that I adored, but they, too, no longer fitted – my life or my feet. Slowly, I put them on eBay or bagged them up ready for a charity shop, bit by bit saying goodbye to my old life.

Believe me when I say that I get how it feels to let go of a previous version of yourself. I get the loss, confusion, pain, sometimes shock, and feeling like the same person on the inside but seeing the face in the mirror changing. It's not just about wrinkles and grey hairs is it? It's what they signify. We know they are a tangible reminder that life is moving on, that nothing lasts for ever. Time clearly isn't standing still and is far more limited than we ever understood when we were younger, feeling invincible.

The realisation hits me every now and then that I'm not part of the young crowd any more. I don't know the music they listen to, I missed when skinny jeans went out of fashion, and I really don't understand how socks with sandals is a thing. When I was away filming with a brilliant team one time, they suggested going out for dinner, which I thought was a great idea. Until they suggested meeting at 9pm. At 9pm?! I'd usually be thinking about heading to bed at that time of night!

On the surface these things are small, but they speak volumes, increasing our sense of loss – that we're no longer part of the group in society that we identified with for years. Youth is so

Time will keep marching on no matter how many face creams we buy.

idolised that we often have to grieve it before we can embrace the good things about our age.

When I was healing and missing my old face, if someone had said to me, 'Just get over it', that wouldn't have helped. If they'd said, 'Don't worry!', that wouldn't have helped. If they'd said, 'Your new face is just as good as your old face', that wouldn't have helped. If they'd tried to hide all the photos and videos and pretend the old me never even existed, that wouldn't have helped either. I needed to grieve.

There can be such huge pressure to be positive all the time that it can become toxic. We prize happiness and, despite growing trends for more honesty on social media, the vast majority of posts are still about people having a wonderful time on holiday or telling the world how much they love their spouse. (I get that – popping on to Instagram to tell the world your spouse really pisses you off probably won't do much to improve the quality of your relationship.) So, talking about ageing in a positive way can become yet another burden that is put on women: 'Don't worry!', 'It's fine!', 'Embrace your wrinkles!', 'Enjoy your grey hairs!' It can be utterly exhausting.

Generally, modern society isn't set up to allow us to grieve – certainly not in many communities in the UK, where there's been a 'stiff upper lip' mentality for so long. We think we should 'put a brave face on it' and 'put our best foot forward'. There is a time and place for that, but trying to move on quickly doesn't always help. It's not realistic and can leave us feeling crap about ourselves. Denying that we feel sad about something doesn't actually mean we feel less sad.

Psychologist Susan David speaks brilliantly about the emotions we don't tend to feel comfortable with and so try to pretend that we don't feel them. She wrote a book, *Emotional Agility*, the title being a process that 'isn't about ignoring difficult emotions and thoughts. It's about holding those emotions and thoughts loosely, facing them courageously and compassionately, and then moving past them to make big things happen in your life.'[1]

She encourages us to be curious about our thoughts and emotions, rather than dismissing them, and to see them for what they are. I can be quite hard on myself, so I find this a really helpful reminder to be more compassionate. Feeling sad that your face and body look different doesn't make you a bad person (or a bad feminist), it's an understandable part of life, so be kind to yourself too. As human beings, we find change hard. Life transitions are hard. We like things to be the same, we like to control them, and the changes we see in the mirror remind us that we really can't! Time will keep marching on no matter how many face creams we buy.

Another thing that wouldn't have helped me in my pain would have been endless wallowing in it. I could have spent days and days looking at my old face in photos but, at a certain point, it just wouldn't have done me any good. I had to let go and say goodbye to the old me. I was thankful for what had been, but needed to be real about what was happening in the present. Now, I can say that I was burned, I'm aware of the reality that I look different from the majority of women, but that's OK. I don't need to be the best-looking woman in the room to be OK with myself and feel comfortable in my own skin.

Similarly, with ageing, we know we're getting older. Even if there was no calendar to tell us, we can see the reality that time is passing in the mirror and feel it in our bones. But becoming older doesn't make us less than anyone else, it's not something shameful that needs to be hidden, and we certainly don't need

We don't have to be ecstatic about the idea of ageing; we just need to find a way to accept it and not have it dominate our thoughts or define how we see ourselves.

to be the youngest in the room to feel good about ourselves. We don't have to be *ecstatic* about the idea of ageing; we just need to find a way to accept it and not have it dominate our thoughts or define how we see ourselves.

We'll go on to talk more about some of the wonderful things about getting older, and the many things we gain, in later chapters but, first of all, it is important to let go of the myth that youth is the most prized of all possessions. We need to realise that we have internalised ageism since we were young and recognise it for what it is: unfounded prejudice.

We get bombarded with these messages right from the beginning. As children, we watched Disney princesses, who were always young. Their adversaries were usually older women, such as the wicked stepmother who was jealous of Cinderella's youth and beauty, so kept her downtrodden, using her as a maid, or the evil fairy who curses Sleeping Beauty because her parents did not invite her to the christening. We've seen a thousand romcoms featuring 20-something characters, because romance is for young people. We hear women being dismissed as 'frumpy' and 'mumsy' (of course, there are no male equivalents of these insults), and having 'let themselves go' or 'given up' as they've got older. Repeatedly people say, 'It's not polite to ask a lady her age', as though it's rude because it's a shameful secret that she would, or should, be embarrassed to admit. We read the birthday cards with their endless 'jokes' about being 'over the hill', it all being 'downhill from here', and life being as good as over once you hit 40.

Someone says, 'You don't look your age' and we say, 'Thank you', but it's not really a compliment. It's a statement about their *perception* of what the reality of being that age is. It's so deeply ingrained in us that, even when we realise it's ageist, we still do it.

We've seen women belittled, judged, and put down because of their age in so many ways, it's no wonder that we can feel depressed about getting older. The question is, is our age the problem?

Ashton Applewhite, author of *This Chair Rocks*, says it's not the passage of time that makes getting older so much harder than it has to be, it's ageism. Similarly, having a vagina isn't what makes life harder for women, it's sexism.[2] She says, 'Ageing is not a problem to be fixed, or a disease to be cured. It is a natural, powerful, life-long process that unites us all.'

How differently would we feel if we took this on board? If we recognised how many of our perceptions of ageing are prejudices and saw the truth instead? We need to start holding up our ideas on what it means to be middle-aged or 'old' up to the light.

When you're 16, 40 feels so far away. For many of us, at that age, our parents were in their 40s and their lives seemed so boring compared to the things we were into. They didn't get why we wanted to spend all night on the phone to our mates, and we didn't get why they were repeatedly trying to drag us out for a walk. Now, when you look around at friends your age, what do you see? I see strength, vitality, energy, positivity, life experiences, wisdom. I don't look at them and think they are sad and boring. I totally get now why my parents enjoyed a walk!

Maybe now, teenagers are looking at *us* and judging us as being irrelevant. Does that mean we actually *are* irrelevant? Of course not! Often the problem with ageing is not the reality of it, it's the concepts we've swallowed and held on to about it for so long without examining them. Do we really believe that we are less than we were? When we take a look at ourselves, our skills, and our experiences, do we conclude that we are less valuable to society than when we were in our 20s? What criteria would such judgements be based on?

It's easy to look back at our youth with rose-tinted glasses, but I wouldn't go back to being that person for anything. I would much rather be my current age, with the experience I've gained, the resilience and wisdom I've won by learning from painful trial and error. I am so much more comfortable in my own skin, now that I know who I am and I've made my peace with my good and bad qualities.

So often, historically but also more recently, the perceived benefit of youth for women has been fertility. It's incredible that so many women can conceive and have babies, but it is not the only thing we bring to the world. Far from it.

Ageism has it that there's a cut-off point for everything. Falling in love, starting a new career, taking up a new hobby, being happy. It's nonsense! Age is no barrier to doing any of these and they might be even better if they happen as we reach midlife. I have friends who met and married in their 40s or later and say that their relationships are the best they've ever had. They've done so much maturing, worked out who they are and what they want, and this has enabled them to make better choices about their partners and how they invest in their relationships to make them work. It's also entirely appropriate to go into some careers later in life, such as counselling. A survey by the British Association for Counselling and Psychotherapy (BACP) found that nearly 80 per cent of its members are aged from 45 to 65+.[3] Even things that are biologically true can be turned around. Just because you can't have a baby yourself beyond the menopause doesn't mean that it's impossible to become a mum later in life – you could foster a child or marry someone who has children. We think we age out of so many areas in life, questioning our hair, make-up, outfit choices and more, asking, 'Is this age-appropriate?' Well, do you like it? If you do, then it's appropriate for your age!

It's easy to look back at our youth with rose-tinted glasses, but I wouldn't go back to being that person for anything.

Rather than seeing ageing as a process of losing things, how about we grieve the things we might be saying goodbye to, while also remembering that there will be wonderful new things to say hello to as well! You *can* start a new hobby, learn a new skill, reinvent yourself, and form new relationships at any age – it's only society that tells you you can't.

If we lived in a culture that honoured older people, perhaps we would look in the mirror and rejoice each time we saw signs of ageing. We'd celebrate each new line, knowing that with it would come the respect of those around us. If we destigmatised getting older, the effect would be transformative. We would let a lot of our hang-ups go and recognise that there's no right or wrong way to look at a particular age. We all experience ageing, but that doesn't mean we all age in the same way. Some elements of how we age are up to us as individuals.

We can make all sorts of changes to our appearance, from dying our hair to getting Botox. Personally, I get regular Botox injections, as it helps make-up sit better on my face and gives me a more hydrated look. But, honestly, I think I probably would have had Botox even if it weren't for the effects of the burns. I dye my hair and I get my nails done. I love getting fully made up, so I don't judge anyone else's choices. I love that it's possible to preserve myself to a certain degree, but I also understand there's only so much I can do. The point isn't *what* I do to alter my appearance; the point is that I make peace with the fact that I'm ageing. If I don't learn to let go of the old and embrace the new, I will forever be chasing my tail, trying to achieve something that's impossible: turning back the clock.

It is possible to embrace new versions of yourself, though, I promise you! I'm not saying that I never have down days or times when I feel insecure. Equally, when the sun comes out, you'll find me by the pool in the tiniest bikini I can find, unashamed of anyone seeing my scars, and not feeling any need to cover up. Sometimes people stare and whisper, but I've got to a place where I'm OK with that. If they are looking and judging me, so what? Am I really going to change my life and do things differently just in case they think I look bad? Why is their opinion more important than my own? If I am happy, does it matter what a stranger thinks? My life is about me, not them! I need to live how I want to live, according to my values and what makes me happy. I hold the key to my self-confidence, but if I put it in the hands of others, I will waiver continually depending on who I'm with. So, while I love to get my hair and make-up done, I'm not a slave to my appearance. I will happily go to the gym, do the school run, or jump on Instagram with no make-up and unwashed hair. It doesn't make me less in any way!

I'm not here to tell you that you should or shouldn't do things to change your appearance as you age. It would be totally hypocritical of me! Plus, I'm done with people policing women's bodies. Telling us we shouldn't use things that are deemed anti-ageing is as bad as telling us we should use them. It's your body, your choice. I just want to encourage us all to embrace who we are and to question what's going on when we don't feel comfortable with our ageing body. Do we not like wrinkles in and of themselves or have we been taught to think that they are a bad thing? Are we getting fillers or using expensive elixirs because we want to or we're trying to live up to someone else's impossible standards? Let's think about *why* we do what we do, the narratives we've been fed, and whether we want to continue to believe them or to write our own stories instead. Let's not forget that the women who are held up as 'ageing well' are chosen because the media thinks they look youthful. Also, often they are some of the most beautiful women in the world, so are not an entirely helpful standard for any of us to attempt to set for ourselves. Women such as Eva Mendes, Jennifer Garner, and Victoria Beckham entered their 50s looking amazing, but do they become just another stick for society to beat us with? They're telling us that's how we should or could look when it's not realistic.

No matter what we do, we can't stop the passage of time. We can dye our grey hair, but it doesn't turn back the clock so we're magically 25 again. What we can do, though, is embrace where we're at and make the most of it.

If we're spending time and money we don't have on beauty products and treatments to make us feel better, it may not be because of what we see in the mirror. It's more likely that the problem lies in how we feel inside. The world of beauty products is all artificial but, so long as we realise this and are aware it's a crutch, that's fine. We need to relinquish some control – something, I admit, I'm not very good at!

Something that has helped me is to remember to speak to myself the way I would speak to a friend. I can be so harsh on myself, but I would never criticise a friend's appearance or attack their worth like that. I try to hold on to the thought that I am worthy of the same love and respect I show others. I also find that it's not a good idea to dwell too much on the past. When I went back to my parents' house after being in hospital, my mum had removed all the old pictures of me and that was really helpful. Life keeps moving forward, so you can't spend too much time looking behind you. Of course, I had to have a lot of therapy to help me come to terms with what I'd lost, but I think all of us benefit from being honest about the things we're struggling with.

I'll share more in Chapter 8 about how changing our

perspective and being grateful can make a huge difference to how we feel. For now, though, let me just say that the goal isn't to love every single thing about ageing – that's not realistic. The goal is to accept ourselves where we are. When we hate how we look, we're at war with ourselves and that's precious energy we're using up on the wrong fight. Life is exhausting enough without turning in on yourself. Make peace with your body. Allow yourself to grieve what's gone and say goodbye to what's behind you, so that you have space to embrace all that's ahead. There is so much more to come.

A moment to pause
•••

What will you miss most about your youth? Be kind to yourself as you remember the good and bad that has happened in your life so far, and make peace with the good and bad of life as it is now. What might it feel like to make peace with your body? What's a step you could take towards that?

4

Own your story

One of the things about getting older is that we've racked up a number of life experiences. Some good, some bad, and some that can fill us with shame. I want to look at some of those things that we have found most difficult, some of the biggest challenges we've faced, and how we don't have to let them define us. We can take back control of how a situation serves us, even if that situation was completely out of our control, and something we would never have chosen. Owning my story made me who I am today and I hope I can encourage you to embrace yours, whatever it may be.

As a victim of rape, I was entitled to anonymity in the press. I even considered the offer from the police of going into the witness protection scheme, until I decided that I couldn't leave behind so many people I loved. Because there was no name attached and no story hook for the press, few papers covered the trials. Those that did ran just a paragraph or two of copy about them, buried in among other news. I would forever be 'Girl A' unless I decided to waive my right to anonymity – something that I knew I had to do if I wanted to reclaim my story.

I couldn't conceive of people knowing who I was until the trials were over and I knew whether or not the perpetrators were behind bars. I was on tenterhooks, scared to leave the house alone, frightened every time someone came to the door.

The defendants' lawyers were allowed to take my phone and

trawl through my messages and photos, using anything they liked to paint a picture of me that suited their story. The more promiscuous they could make me out to be, the less likely there was to be a guilty verdict in the rape trial. They used my modelling career against me, that I'd been confident and outgoing, had previous boyfriends – anything they thought would help them. It felt as though I was the one on trial, not my attackers. Day after day they built a story of a woman who was unrecognisable to me – even trying to make out that I had been some sort of gangster, which was completely ridiculous.

While they spun their tale in court, I could say nothing. I felt voiceless. I couldn't fight back and tell them the truth about who I was and what I'd been through because the courts don't work like that. I had to wait for an opportunity for my barrister to shift the focus where it belonged – on to those who were on trial.

Few of us would argue that the courts are now totally safe places for women who are victims of sexual assault, but back then it was even worse. It was only a few years before that the law acknowledged rape could happen between a husband and wife – a wedding ring is not a sign of permanent consent. The culture then was heavily biased towards blaming the victim in such cases. What had she done wrong? Had she been on her own? In the wrong part of town? Was she wearing a short skirt? Had too much to drink? Had multiple previous partners? As though any of these things mean it is your fault that a man violates you. If you knew the man (and one study has found that more than 90 per cent of rape and sexual assault victims do),[1] and if you'd previously had a consensual sexual encounter with him, it was even harder to get a conviction.

The prevalence of the blaming of victims led me to fear that somehow it really was my fault, that somehow I'd brought this on myself and I 'deserved' it. I was filled with shame.

At the same time, my mum was trying to help me get back out into the world around me. My parents' house, where I was staying, had become my safe cocoon and it took a long time and a lot of therapy before I felt able to leave. My acid attack had happened in broad daylight, in a nice area, on a road filled with people, so nowhere felt safe. My mum patiently encouraged me to keep trying. 'We'll just go into town,' she'd say. 'Have a look around some shops for an hour and see how you go.'

I would try to hide myself under a big hat and a mask, but people would still stop and stare, sometimes following us from shop to shop, trying to get a better look. This made me feel self-conscious the whole time and permanently on edge. I knew my mum was right – I couldn't live my life behind closed doors for ever – but the fact that no one had ever seen someone who looked like me didn't make it easy. As well as the stares, people regularly asked us to leave the shop we were in. I had no fight in me to argue. I just wanted to disappear.

One day, as we walked down the road, a white van approached us from behind. From the back, I looked like lots of other girls, so the driver would have presumed that I was a pretty young woman with long blonde hair. I heard the wolf whistle and cringed. Seconds later, as the van drove past, the lecherous driver glimpsed my face and his expression changed to a grimace. His face then filled with disgust and he threw the sandwich he was holding straight at me. Bits of bacon, lettuce, and tomato landed in my hair and stuck to my clothes. I felt totally humiliated.

I let out a scream. It wasn't just about him; I was done. Done with being disfigured, done with being made to feel repulsive, done with feeling like I was utterly worthless. I wanted to shout,

'I am not this person!' All people could see was the outside and they were making snap judgements based purely on that. I felt like I had no voice. Who would take the time to listen to me? To find out not only what had happened that left me looking like this but also who I was – who I really was on the inside.

A few people had already suggested that I document my journey of recovery, but I wasn't sure how much there was to tell. Over time, I slowly warmed to the idea and began filming myself on an old camcorder (phones didn't have video functions then).

A friend said that they would introduce me to a journalist who might be interested in my story and my parents and I discussed at length whether I should call him. It would mean waiving my right to anonymity. It wasn't an easy decision to make and we all had our concerns and fears. Would it be safe? Would people judge me and say that it was my fault? Would I be made to feel even more disgusting than I already did? There were so few disabled or disfigured people in the public eye at that time. There weren't visibly different TV presenters, stars of ad campaigns, or contestants on the line-up of *Strictly Come Dancing* and other TV programmes like we (thankfully) have now. I didn't want to be pitied and I wasn't looking for sympathy; I just wanted to have a voice. I wanted people to see past how I looked to the real me. I wanted to stop being pigeonholed as 'the girl who was attacked' and for people to see that I was a fully rounded, multifaceted human being, just like them.

When I did decide to meet the journalist my friend had mentioned, he was a decent and kind man. After I shared my story he said, 'This is much more than a news piece; it's a much bigger story than that. It needs to be a documentary or book.' He made some introductions and I ended up speaking to some people who were interested in these ideas. It was the team behind Channel 4's *Cutting Edge* documentary series that made me feel the most comfortable. I'd be working with two women – one directing, one shooting – and there was no pressure to do anything I didn't want to do. They weren't going to sensationalise the story or push a particular narrative; they just wanted to film me over the course of a year and see how things developed.

We got on really well from the start and became close. My world was so small at that point and I saw them more than anyone else except my closest family and friends. They came with me to doctors' appointments, filmed me during and after surgery, came to France, where I had non-surgical treatments, and accompanied me to meetings with the police and lawyers. They also documented what day-to-day life looked like for me at home with my family. They were the first people I'd trusted outside those in my immediate circle and I felt comfortable letting them see everything. There was no make-up, no special lighting to try to hide anything, just me. If I was going to show my face to the world, I might as well do it properly.

While we were filming, my attitude had been, 'What's the worst that can happen?' I was already being asked to leave places, having doors slammed in my face, and stuff thrown at me. I knew, too, that the members of the team cared about me and my story – I couldn't have been in safer hands. But, the night before the documentary was due to air, suddenly I panicked. I was worried that I'd made a mistake and I should have stayed anonymous. Once the programme went out, there would be no taking it back and I was petrified that someone who saw it would decide to attack me.

The next day, the director called to tell me that the programme had been watched by 3.5 million people. Such was my state of mind, I assumed she meant that they'd had 3.5 million complaints. I was so convinced this was what was waiting for me, I couldn't

There's something so powerful about showing the world the real you, in your most vulnerable and raw state, and being met with kindness.

comprehend that so many people had tuned in to find out about my story. My fears vanished as the response was overwhelmingly positive. In the weeks following, post began arriving and, eventually, I filled three ring binders with letters. I've kept each piece of correspondence to this day as they still mean so much to me.

I'd been exposed to the horrors of humanity, the lowest people could go, but having told my story and shown the reality of what I was dealing with on camera, I met with the best of humanity. There was love and kindness, people sending prayers and blessings or offering the best bits of advice they knew. Many simply encouraged me to keep going and said they wished me all the best for the future. A number of transgender people contacted me saying they understood the feeling I'd expressed of being stuck behind a façade that you don't feel represents who you are, but you can't get people to see beyond it. I had letters from women and men who had been raped saying, 'This happened to me too.' Each word of kindness, each person saying 'Me too' healed a little piece of me. My soul had been so violated, to the point it was almost destroyed, but now I was making connections with wonderful people and those connections were healing more and more of me. They gave me the confidence to continue and encouraged me to believe that I would make it through.

There's something so powerful about showing the world the real you, in your most vulnerable and raw state, and being met with kindness. It was like breathing out after holding it in for the longest time. Maybe I could show up in the world, even after all I'd been through. Maybe there really was a place for me in it.

Despite the kind letters I had received and this increase in my confidence, I was still nervous about how the wider public would react to me. When I ventured back to the shops with my mum after the documentary had aired, people again approached us and I held my breath thinking that they were about to ask us to leave like before. Instead, they said that they had watched the programme and wanted to wish us well. I could have cried with relief. I'd felt like an alien for a year, like I was in a world that didn't have room for me, but suddenly people were budging up and shifting over to make space for me to sit down.

Let me assure you, there's space for you, too, whatever you've been through or are going through. For so long, women have simply accepted the cultural norms that there are certain things you don't talk about, especially things like periods, hormones, fertility, and the menopause. It's crazy to think that we've been silenced and left to struggle alone all this time when literally half the population faces these issues! I've loved seeing how so many women have started talking about menopause. When I turned 30, it still felt like an unknown, strange secret that meant many of us were clueless about what it might entail, except the cliché of the occasional hot flush that had been the butt of many jokes over the years. I'm so grateful to all the women who have shared their stories, done extensive research, and raised their voices to help those of us who are coming up behind them to not feel alone, and become informed. Our mothers would have had limited options for help with understanding the symptoms of menopause and perimenopause. We can take our pick – doctors run clinics, workplaces offer seminars, and there are countless books, articles, documentaries, podcasts, social media content, and other sources that cover everything we could ever possibly want to know. We might still have a way to go, but the key message is that this isn't something we need to deal with alone – we can be prepared and have places and people we can turn to, whatever our symptoms and experiences may be.

I wish I'd known what a difference not keeping quiet about

it but telling my story could make when I took my first, tentative, steps back out into the world after the attack. As I look back, I still credit the public for the life I now lead. If I hadn't opened up and received such a warm response, chances are that I would have remained a recluse, living something that vaguely resembled a life, but hiding in the shadows, fearful of how I would be received everywhere I went. The world had felt so dangerous to me that I'd shunned it for the best part of eight months. After the programme, I came to see how gentle, kind, and loving people can be and it woke me up and drew me back out into the world.

As sharing my own story was so powerful, I admire others who share theirs, so I provide an opportunity for them to do so on my social media account. Ana got in touch with me in 2021, two years after she was first diagnosed with HIV, to share her story on my Instagram account. When the nurse told her she was HIV positive, she couldn't stop crying, even when she was reassured that HIV was no longer a death sentence and, with medication, it wouldn't be life-limiting. She said, 'The second nurse I saw that day was judgemental and stigmatised me. It was then I realised, this condition wasn't going to kill me but the stigma attached to it could. With my diagnosis came depression, anxiety, panic attacks, and suicidal thoughts. I went on to meet some amazing healthcare professionals who couldn't have been better allies to those of us living with HIV, but my experience shows how someone's attitude can have a huge detrimental impact on us.' Ana shared her story anonymously and, at that time, the only people she'd told about her condition other than medical practitioners and the HIV community were her children and three close friends. She had also started an anonymous Instagram account and posted: 'I slowly accepted that I couldn't

We can't fight what's gone before. The only thing we can do is pour our energy into what happens next. The future is in our hands.

change what had happened to me but I could own my story and be part of the fight against HIV.'

Ana was met with such kindness by people who follow my social media account. So many people thanked her for her vulnerability and courage in sharing her story. They wished her well, sent their love, shared their own stories, offered help, told her how much they respected her, and that she was an inspiration. Some shared how they wished they could convince those they love with HIV that they have nothing to be ashamed of.

Ana was blown away by the response. It helped her to feel more confident and accepting of her situation, and realise that she wasn't defined by her HIV diagnosis. Seeing people's respect for her and kindness gave her the strength she needed to share the news with other significant people in her life, including her mother, members of her extended family, friends, and her manager. She said, 'I am a healthcare professional who has never looked down on people living with HIV but, once I was facing the stigma myself, I was ashamed and feared judgement. By opening up, I felt relieved and the shame and fear faded away. When I started to talk, I started to live again. I found myself again. I could drop my mask and now I'm living an authentic and empowered life.

'To anyone else who feels stuck behind the stigma of something that has happened in their life but is considering talking to people about it, I would say there's no rush, do it in your own time when you feel ready. You don't need to tell the full story, just the parts that you feel comfortable to share. There are parts of my story that still need to be told and I still want to tell but it isn't the right time yet. Try not to imagine scenarios of how someone will react. There is no way of knowing this before it happens and these expectations of negative responses are just the stigma playing on our minds. No matter how it goes, you should be proud of yourself and your story, and how much you have overcome.'

Ana has gone on to be an advocate for those living with HIV, working with George House Trust and sharing her journey on Instagram (@herinvisibledifference). It's incredible to see her powerfully sharing her story to inspire and support others to thrive while living with HIV.

There are lots of things in our lives that can cause us to feel shame and make us want to hide the truth from others. There's a very real, very human, fear that, if people really knew the truth about us, they would look at us differently, judge us harshly, or not want to be around us. But Brené Brown, an author and researcher who studies courage, vulnerability, and shame, says it's only by owning what has happened to us that we can stop them from limiting us. As she says, 'When we deny our stories, they define us. When we own our stories, we get to write a brave new ending.'[2]

I love that empowering message: we get to decide what happens from here. As I said, we all have baggage of some kind or another, whether it's stuff from our childhood or something that's happened more recently. It could be our lack of education, the abuse we've been subjected to, a stutter, infertility, a feeling of failure regarding our work or romantic life, a physical impediment, the breakdown of a relationship with a friend, partner, or family member… The list goes on. Shame isolates us and tries to keep us hiding in the shadows, but owning our story means we have a chance to change it. We can't fight what's gone before. The only thing we can do is pour our energy into what happens next. The future is in our hands.

If your life were a book or a film, you'd likely be in the middle

You are never too old to write your own story.

of the timespan, which can often feel a bit messy. Chances are, there have been chapters of good and bad stuff but, either way, the story isn't over yet. If you were writing the book, would you have the protagonist hide away in shame? Stay stuck in her past, defined by one thing and perhaps live a smaller life because of it? Or would you find a way to change the narrative, bring something good out of something bad, and show people that stereotypes are lazy and don't help anyone?

I felt that my burns were defining what people thought about me and I wanted to take back the right to define myself. Likewise, you are not defined by one thing. We like to label stuff. 'Oh, she's a single mum.' 'She's depressed.' 'She's divorced.' 'She's single.' 'She's a stay-at-home mum.' 'She's academic.' 'She's autistic.' 'She's a career woman.' Nobody is one thing alone! We can't be summed up by one label, no matter how much more convenient that would be for other people!

What I didn't know beforehand was that sharing my story would empower other people to share theirs. Not just burns and sexual assault survivors, but all sorts of people who could relate to feeling labelled and stuck, isolated, and alone. Me putting myself out there on TV, without hiding or trying to neaten the story to make it into something more palatable, helped them feel seen. This was not that easy or common at the time, but we have seen it more and more since the advent of social media. Women now share their stories of things that previous generations kept hidden, like the realities of chemotherapy and the ravages of cancer, what it's like using a colostomy bag, the highs and lows of blending families post a divorce, or how it feels to live with an addiction. Social media provides a space where people can open up and, in doing so, make themselves and others feel less alone.

That said, going public isn't for everyone and I'm in no way suggesting we all go around telling everyone loads of personal details about our lives. Social media isn't always a safe place and not all of us want to share things with the world. The point isn't to share it widely, it's simply to share it. This could be with only one or two people you love and trust. It's not about numbers, it's about being known. I couldn't have trusted my story to just anyone when I agreed to do the documentary. I was so incredibly vulnerable and could have been at the mercy of how the producers wanted to portray me. They could have sensationalised my story and painted me a particular way and I knew that once it was out there, there was no way to take it back. But once I'd found the right team, I was so glad I'd shown the real me. It meant that I knew I was accepted for who I was, not for what people saw on the surface. The whole experience and reactions to the programme gave me true confidence, of a kind that was much deeper than I'd ever had, even before I was attacked. The ground on which my life was then based felt firmer because I no longer believed that people would accept me only if they didn't find out certain things about me or I looked a certain way. It gave me permission to be my authentic self, and that has run through my life ever since. I haven't felt like I need to hide or to pretend that I'm totally on top of everything. I'm always keen in my books, interviews, and on social media to be real and honest. What's the point in pretending otherwise? People can only accept me properly if they actually know me. And if they reject me? That's their decision and I'll be fine. I've lived through worse.

Over the years, people have called me inspirational and while that's a lovely compliment and something I hugely appreciate, I'm not sure it's true. People imagine that from day one I was bouncing back and throwing myself into rebuilding my life. The truth is, it was a long, hard road. I was glad the documentary showed how fearful I was, as well as the times when I was joking and trying to lighten the mood. It showed that there were moments when I didn't see any point to my life, as well as ones when I was celebrating with friends and family about how far I'd come. That's the reality, not a sugar-coated pseudo-inspirational version of it. Even when the documentary came out and I had got to a point where I was able to live on my own, I was still seriously struggling. People saw me as being brave, but I was still scared and in a lot of pain – physically and emotionally. I was sent bottles of champagne by people congratulating me on the documentary, but I didn't drink them with friends, toasting how wonderful life was. I was drinking them alone, desperate for something that would help me sleep and blot out the pain. Trying to make my way in the world was exhausting.

I hope my story does inspire people, but I don't want that to be because I've presented myself as someone who has it all together, who never gets down. I have my good days and bad days. Days when I can't believe how far I've come and feel like I could conquer the world, and days when I weep on the stairs, wishing I was six years old and someone would come along and take care of everything for me. That's life. Anyone who tells you they have everything under control 24/7 is lying.

Sharing my story helped to broaden my perspective too. When we go through hard stuff we naturally become more focused on ourselves because we're trying to find a way to deal with it. I felt as though I was one of the first people who looked like me, who had experienced what had happened to me, to make themselves visible on TV, and what I found was that others were suffering in similar ways and maybe there was a way I could do something to help them. The joy of helping people was a tonic for me at a time when I felt so helpless in very many ways. Just by being vulnerable, people said it was making a difference to their life and that amazed me.

All that happened from then on became the start of a new story for me, and I want to offer this to you as you consider how to embrace the years that are ahead of you. The attack and the recovery weren't the ending for me; they were the middle. As I owned my story, I gave myself the ability to write the kind of ending that I wanted. You can do this too. Whatever you've been through in the past, it doesn't have to be what defines you as you move forward. You get to choose, you get to create the life you want, and you don't have to let the hardest bits be the things that shape your future. You may well be a product of your past, but you don't have to be a prisoner of it and, no matter what has happened, there is life ahead. You are never too old to write your own story. There is hope. There is more for you.

A moment to pause
●●●

Which part of your story do you find it difficult to make peace with? How could you rewrite the ending so it's something you're proud of?

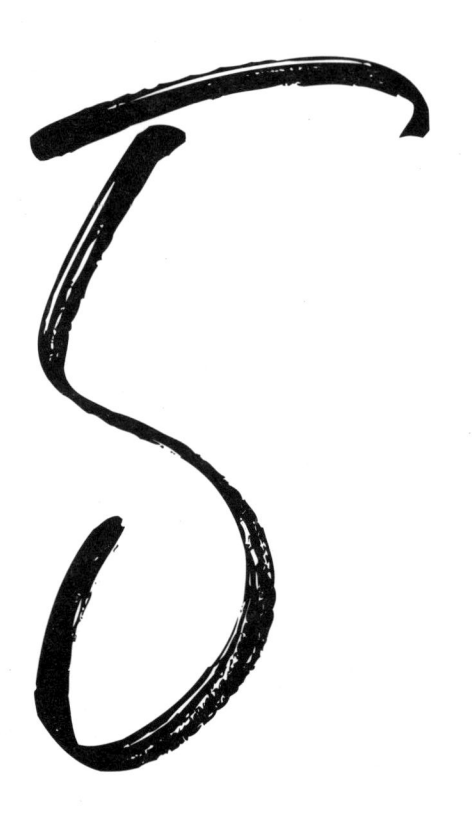

Finding purpose

What am I here for? It's a question many of us ask ourselves, especially around middle age. Some of the amazing responses I'd had, and the things I was discovering about my true value and self-worth, felt like secrets that should be shared with the world and I wanted to do that. This led me down a new path of looking at what made me feel alive and asking the big questions about who I am and what I'm here for.

Looking back, I consider myself fortunate to have discovered my purpose when I did as I realise that, often, it's something people only discover much later in life. We can be busy and distracted by so many things but, without a sense of purpose, we can feel lost or unfocused, finding that days, weeks, months, years, drift by and we haven't grasped what we want to do with our life, and time is precious. No one wants to wake up at 80 and realise that they have wandered aimlessly through their days, never making the most of life or understanding the impact they could have made. We want to find our purpose and act on it as soon as we can.

At outpatient clinics, I would see a lot of other burns survivors and I realised that I looked different from them. Living in the UK, we'd all received the same acute care from the National Health Service (NHS), but additional treatments I'd been privileged to have in France had made a huge difference, not only to how I looked but also, more importantly, to movements I could make. They'd enabled me to blink, turn my head, and regain the use of my mouth – all key functions that have a major impact on quality of life.

These differences made me want better physical outcomes for all people who are recovering from burns. I was desperate, too, for them to know that there is life after a burn injury. I saw so many people who had lost hope and didn't know how to make their way in the world after they were injured. I knew what it was like – I'd been in the same position. The only people I'd seen who had scars like mine outside these clinics were those whose images were used by charities for fundraising. Often, they were armed forces veterans, so their experiences were very different from mine and those of many burns survivors I met. I didn't need people to feel sorry for me and I was learning that I didn't need to make myself less or hide away. I wanted more for all those who had been through something similar to me.

The documentary I mentioned in Chapter 4 had given me a rare platform and, truthfully, I became a bit manic in my desire to make the most of it to share this amazing hope that I'd found! I'd spent a long time thinking 'Why me?' about the attack, but now I began to think, 'Why not me?' There was also something else that had happened and it motivated me.

I seriously considered taking my own life not long after the attack, but had an experience that stopped me. I can only attribute it to God, even though I'd not previously been religious and am not from a religious family. I was alone in my hospital room when I started feeling warm and bright, and suddenly I knew that there was going to be a life for me beyond this. It was like hearing a voice that said, 'There's a reason to live. If you kill yourself, you'll be missing out.' Perhaps the reason to keep going was that I could help other people because of what I'd been through.

My parents were on board with me starting a charity and helped me set up a bank account specifically for it, with the help also of an incredible person I met while I was working on the documentary for Channel 4. I had to borrow the money required to start my charity as I wasn't able to work because I was still in the intensive phase of my recovery so had no income.

Something amazing started happening. When people heard my story, they wanted to give me money. I was living at home rent free and receiving benefits so I definitely couldn't keep the money for myself. People would also offer things like nice holidays for me to go on, but I was still too unwell to do anything like that so, every time someone offered some kind of help, I would tell them that they could do so by paying a donation into the bank account instead.

My only plan for the charity at the start was for it to be a fund that could enable burns survivors to receive treatment at the rehab centre in France that had helped my recovery so much. But the money kept on coming, and it was way more than we needed to realise that vision. Then TV presenter and entrepreneur Simon Cowell got in touch, which was not something I would have ever imagined happening! He'd seen my documentary and said he wanted to help. Initially he offered me a job at his production company, which in itself made me realise how much things had changed for me. Rather than bite his hand off and grasp the opportunity, I told him that what I really wanted to do was change things for burns survivors. Amazingly, he said he'd get behind me and I knew that having him on board would change the charity's reach considerably.

Up until then, we'd been doing things a bit haphazardly. Initially, I ran the charity from my bedroom at my parents' house on a dodgy old laptop that was infuriatingly slow. When I was able to live independently again and get a flat in London, I would meet up with women burns survivors I met through the charity. Local hairdressing salons let me use their premises on Sundays when they were closed and I would do the women's hair, make-up, and nails. I taught them how to achieve the looks themselves and use make-up effectively, passing on everything I'd been learning about how to deal with my own scars. Other beauticians began to volunteer their time, seeing what a difference these sessions made to the women, helping them regain their self-confidence.

As the scope of the charity began to change, we needed to become more professional and appoint a board of trustees. I had never had an office job, so I didn't have a clue how to do half the things that were now coming up. I'm not exaggerating when I say that I had to Skype my sister to find out how to reload a stapler so I could attach the sheets of the trustees paperwork together! Amazingly, lots of people offered me their time, expertise, and resources, and that in itself was healing for me. Before the attack, I'd always felt that any offers from men were made because they wanted something in exchange. Now men, and women, were going out of their way to help without the expectation of anything in return.

It was all fully outside my comfort zone. I even had to learn how to dress myself appropriately for work so that nothing interfered with the feeding tube I still needed at the time. I wanted to be able to take pride in my appearance and maintain my dignity, so I found ways to work around it.

Part of my role as CEO of the charity involved standing up in front of the trustees and pitching my ideas – something I'd never done before. More than this, because of the attack, I had to build my ability to trust people again and be confident enough to make eye contact with them. Just months earlier I'd been too scared to leave the house alone, but now I had a sense of purpose, a reason to get up in the morning. I'm not pretending that drive wiped everything else away – I was still experiencing depression and dealing with trauma – but the structure of being in an office at a certain time each day, with trustees, colleagues, and beneficiaries depending on me, meant I couldn't stay at home in my pyjamas. It changed my life as well as the lives of the people we were trying to support in their own recovery.

However, ultimately, as the charity continued to grow, it became too much for me. All the emails and requests came to me and it was overwhelming spending all day every day hearing people's traumatic stories when I was still processing my own trauma. I wanted to do it but the charity was taking over my life and it wasn't sustainable, so we recruited a new CEO, which enabled me to step back and become a trustee rather than be responsible for everything.

Since then, the charity has gone from strength to strength and I'm so proud of the work it does. We now have a team of professionals who are experts in their various fields based at our own residential treatment centre in St Helens, Merseyside, where we provide physical, psychological, and emotional inpatient support. Another large team of voluntary and paid members of staff, including burns survivors, give support to the family members and carers of those with burns. I am still heavily involved with fundraising, raising awareness of the charity, and work with burn survivors, mentoring and advising them, but am able to leave running all the day-to-day aspects in other people's capable hands. It's a privilege for me to work with the people who come to us for help and see them overcome obstacles, reclaim their lives, and find hope and confidence as they move forward. It's the most rewarding and fulfilling part of my professional life.

At the point when I realised that I couldn't carry on being the CEO of the charity as it grew, I also realised that we don't find one purpose in life and that's it. Our purpose can change, expand, and grow as we get older and find ourselves with new experiences and skills, living in new circumstances. Sometimes we find ourselves going back to things we tried years earlier, but with fresh eyes and greater wisdom. Sometimes we'll be surprised to find our purpose lies in something we could never have imagined it would years before. We never know how or when the skills and experiences we're picking up as we go along might come into play.

The charity opened my eyes to the kinds of things I could do and that I was able to make a difference to the lives of other people, while also finding fulfilment myself. I realised that I didn't have to go and find the next project, but I did want to start living with purpose each day, finding the things I was passionate about and living intentionally. It's so easy to let life happen to us, to be so swept up in the everyday that we forget to look at the big picture of who we are and what we bring to the world.

It can feel like we've been on a treadmill since birth. Our direction dictated by school, perhaps further education, the need to get a job – any job – to keep ourselves afloat and, for many, starting a family and all the demands that places on women, physically, mentally, and emotionally. There isn't always a lot of time to work out what we want life to look like. Some of us realise as we get older that life hasn't worked out as we'd hoped. There are those who pursued a creative career and found that

Sometimes we'll be surprised to find our purpose lies in something we could never have imagined it would years before.

the cruel reality is, you can be incredibly talented and still not find a way to make a sustainable living out of it. Others who longed to be a mother, found that it wasn't as easy to get pregnant as the lessons at school led us to believe or, if they did, it wasn't as fulfilling as they believed it would be. Some who had a sense of purpose from a young age – wanting to work as a health care professional, lawyer, accountant – found themselves experiencing burnout and asking, 'Is this it?'

At school, we may have had careers advisers and lots of people ask us what we want to do at that stage but, as an adult, those conversations don't happen unless we instigate them. When are we to find the time to do that, in between the million other demands placed on us? Many of us are juggling varied demands – caring for children, parents, staying on top of everything at work, trying to stay healthy physically, and dealing with a never-ending pile of life admin. My encouragement in response to that would be, we need to value ourselves and what we bring to the world enough to make time and space to really think about our purpose. We all have something that we contribute to this world and we've got too many years ahead of us to not do this. Let's ask the questions!

Clinical psychologist Dr Julie Smith says that people often start therapy when they feel a bit lost and they're not quite sure why. The underlying problem, she says, is that they have disconnected from their core values. She explains: 'Values are not a set of actions that can be completed. Values are a set of ideas about *how* you want to live your life, the *kind* of person you want to be and the *principles* you want to stand for.'[1]

I find Dr Smith's words so helpful when I think about how I want my life to look. 'What do you do?' is probably the question most people ask when meeting someone new and this tells us something about what society values in us – not who we *are* but what we *do*. The next most likely questions women in their 30s and onwards are asked are, of course, 'Are you married?' and 'Do you have kids?' Something that drives me so mad is the emphasis put on us to have a partner and procreate. We will come back to it in Chapter 6. Wouldn't we have more interesting conversations if we asked, 'What are you passionate about?' or 'What makes you happy?' The answers people give might relate back to their paid employment and their choices to marry and have children or they might not.

The values and principles Dr Smith is referring to are unique to you. If you try to borrow someone else's, you'll find it a slog to live by the things that are important to them rather than what's really important to you. I often get up at 5am to exercise and people tell me that's crazy. I get it – it's not for everyone. For me, having been in a coma and lost so much physical strength, it's hugely important to me to keep my body strong. My diary is so often full, if I want to exercise, that's the best time of day to make it happen. But my value of prioritising my health is no more noble or worthwhile than another woman's values of rest and her choosing to sleep until 8am because, for her, that is one of the ways she achieves her value of nourishing her body.

It's also important to me to put in my diary times when I volunteer in women's prisons. I was invited to a prison a number of years ago to speak to some women who had been victims of domestic violence. Just like setting up the charity, it was outside my comfort zone to do this, not knowing what to expect or what I could offer. I came away excited and inspired by the women I met and the conversations we'd had, keen to continue volunteering and supporting women in prison, which I've done ever since. Despite all I've been through, I don't believe that there are bad people. I think people end up in bad circumstances and make bad choices. Not everyone understands why I would want to devote time to doing this but, for me, it helps make sense of my past. If I can do something to support and help these women, I will. I know that my response and the connection my volunteering has to my values will not be shared by everyone who has been a victim of crime and I fully respect that.

If you've never had time to think about what your core values are, you can find loads of free resources online that list lots of possible values to help you work out what's really important to you. They can help you think through questions such as: 'Is it important to you to be adventurous in your life? Reliable? Kind? Independent? Creative? Spiritual? Courageous? Authentic?' It could be all these things! There are no right or wrong answers and, even within each value, interpretations will vary from person to person.

Whatever values we discover, they will vary during our life as they can change with our circumstances and age. My strong work ethic has looked vastly different in the various seasons of my life. As soon as I got my National Insurance number at the age of 16, I started working as a cleaner before school. Then I went on to work in my local supermarket, taking as many evening and weekend shifts as I could.

When I was recovering after the acid attack, it seemed like there was so little I could do, so little I could control, and I couldn't work, so I decided to put everything into my recovery, treating it as though it were my job. I would dress up for hospital appointments and make sure I was always on time. I built good relationships with those in the medical teams helping me, like they were my colleagues. Doing this provided me with a little community and I realised that, as I invested in other people, caring about what was important to them, they became invested in me too. I became so close to my surgeon that he became a good friend to me and my parents, to the extent that we're in touch all these years later and I was a guest at his daughter's wedding.

I'd never been a writer before but I found that keeping a journal during my recovery was really helpful, and I started writing a blog for my family. I was still barely able to see at that point, but I kept it up, like I was being paid for it. I started writing my story into a book, even though I had no idea if I'd ever be able to find a publisher. Every Friday, it gave me a reason to get showered, dressed, and take a photocopy of my manuscript with a covering letter addressed to a publisher and head to my local post office. Years later, during the Covid pandemic, when TV work wasn't possible, I used a lot of the time this gave me to work on my house, painting all the skirting boards and having 'design meetings' with my family when we planned renovations.

All these expressions of my work ethic helped me to find meaning at times when I needed it and enabled me to throw myself into them with all the energy I had. They weren't all paid employment, but they helped me to feel like me, often in situations that were as far from ideal as you can get. We can't control our circumstances, but our values can help guide us when things feel out of control.

They can be more helpful than goals, as many factors can affect whether or not they are achieved. Growing up, my goals were to have a career in TV and modelling, then get married and have kids. I'd picked up on all society's cues that told me my happiness and purpose would be found in marriage and motherhood, so was waiting to meet what I heard would be my 'other half'. When my life changed so radically, I couldn't conceive that would still happen. In part, I couldn't imagine anyone wanting to marry me, because I'd also understood that I needed to look a certain way to find a husband. I was also no longer sure I wanted a man in my life after what had happened to me at the hands of two men. I knew that I had to let go of my original goal and try to find fulfilment outside a romantic relationship.

When I look back, before the attack I was only really interested in short-term gratification. I wanted attention and I think my life was heading in a sad direction. The world I was inhabiting was shallow and self-serving and I wonder whether I would have ended up going down some dark paths in my search for continual highs. Nearly dying changed my understanding of life and how precious it is. Helping people through my documentary and charity led to me seeing how much can be gained not from what we take but from what we give.

I've heard it said that you find your purpose in life by looking at how your passions can serve the world. A word of warning: as women, we're often programmed to give, to put ourselves last on the list and make sure everyone else's needs are met before we even think about our own. That's not the type of giving I'm talking about. I'm talking about giving in ways that make us feel alive, things that give us a sense of purpose and bring their own rewards.

There are a couple of other things I'm wary of when we talk about purpose. The first is that it might make you think that it has to be a something huge, but it doesn't. We're not talking about a generation-defining artistic masterpiece, a significant scientific breakthrough, or an act of courage that means you have a statue erected in your honour. For most of us, purpose is about small, everyday things, like being a good daughter, sister,

Helping people through my documentary and charity led to me seeing how much can be gained not from what we take but from what we give.

friend, colleague, parent, neighbour. It's about living in our values wherever we find ourselves spending our time each day. It doesn't have to be pressured or make the headlines to be worthwhile.

The second thing I hate is the idea that living with purpose means you're active and focused on it 24/7. That's not real life! To me, the 'girl boss' mentality, the superwoman ideal, and the myth that we can 'have it all' are really unhelpful. I try to achieve a lot in my life but no one can smash their goals every single day. We all have down days, times we're tired or ill, seasons when our mental health requires us to make a bit more time to rest. We all question what we're doing with our lives sometimes and whether we're good at anything. We don't need to run ourselves into the ground every day to prove we're worthy. We need to be real about the struggles we have trying to balance everything we've got going on. And we need to remember there's a place for watching crap TV! You're not failing if you're aware of your own needs and take a break. Exhaustion and burnout are bad for our physical, mental, and emotional wellbeing; they're not badges of honour we should be clamouring for.

Mothers are often made to feel bad for not being at school sports days because they're working, or for not having as successful a career as they could because they work part-time to be around for their kids. And women who decide not to have children or who aren't able to? That's a whole separate category of judgement. It feels like we're always being compared to other women making different choices or facing different circumstances and found wanting. We're set up to fail because you can't do it all. And while we're talking about this, the same pressures are not applied to men. Even with how far we've got in terms of equality, the Fatherhood Institute found that men only spend 65 per cent of the time women do on childcare, and that's with Covid accounting for 18 per cent of the increase on the previous figure, which was prior to the pandemic.[2] One study of more than 200,000 people in ten different countries found that women spend 70 minutes more per day than their male partners doing household chores like cleaning, washing clothes, and prepping meals.[3] In same-sex relationships, the division tends to be more equal.[4]

So many of us are trying to balance everything with this extra load but then we see people on Instagram talking about how their freelance career has taken off, the incredible DIY they're doing on their homes, the perfect family life they're leading, or huge friendship group they keep up with. Let's not compare ourselves to each and every story and then assume that we're lacking. No one person can do everything! We need to be honest about that with one another or we set ourselves up to fail.

I'm aware that I often try to pack too much into my life and it can be difficult for the people around me to deal with that. It's made me successful in some areas of my life, but if I'm not careful, it can damage my relationships. When I'm intentional about how I want to spend my life, and not just caught up in the busyness of day-to-day life, I step back and realise that I need more balance and I'm the only one who can make that happen. It helps me to focus on how I want to be in the future and take steps towards living like that.

If we carry this sense of living intentionally and by our values, it will serve us well in all aspects of our life as we get older. If we don't – and we make one thing our identity – we will struggle when life moves on. Getting so caught up in motherhood that we don't experience a sense of purpose in other areas of our life too may mean it's very difficult to let our kids grow up and become less reliant on us. Making work our focus may mean that when there are times we can't work, due to illness, redundancy, or – ultimately – when we retire, we feel lost. If we grasp who we are and what we bring to the world, we can carry that with us always, at any age, any life stage, and in any circumstance. You have a unique combination of gifts and passions to bring to the world, so don't hold back.

A moment to pause
●●●

Rather than asking yourself, 'What do I want to do?', ask yourself, 'Who do I want to be?' Take some time to consider what your values are and how they show you more about your purpose.

6

Happily ever after?

When we are looking at finding our sense of purpose, it can often feel like all our youth is building towards us meeting our ideal romantic partner and becoming mothers, as though that is the entire reason for our existence. There's seemingly little thought given to what happens after you meet that person and have walked off into the sunset. What if the relationship turns out not to keep to the 'till death us do part' bit. What if you don't meet that person in the first place.

It strikes me that all the pressure involved is one of the reasons why midlife can feel like a bit of a wasteland and ageing can be terrifying. We'll talk about this later in this chapter, but the sense that our purpose is to get married and have children can make it feel like there's little to look forward to once we've hit those milestones, and life can only go downhill afterwards, or we're flailing around with nothing to look forward to if we haven't. As I said in Chapter 5, romance and parenthood aren't the only reasons we're put on this planet, but I understand the pressures people experience and idealistic standards related to them only too well. Let me explain how I came to understand by telling you what I had to put up with when I started pursuing the idea of meeting someone perfect for me.

Dating isn't for the faint-hearted at the best of times, but when I was first stepping back into the dating pool following the attack, it was definitely not the best of times. I moved back to London after recovering at my parents' house, was living in a flat, and slowly regaining my social life and starting to see friends again. For a long time after the attack I had let go of the idea of getting married. Healing from what had happened, keeping up with hospital appointments, and rebuilding my strength were more than enough to be getting on with. But now I wanted to go out to bars with friends, I wanted to regain my confidence, and I was feeling ready to meet a guy.

It was a minefield. I would try to style my hair so it covered as much of my burned skin as I could, but most bars had very subdued lighting, so men often didn't notice my injuries at first. I would drink more than I should to make me feel more confident, but then, if we exchanged numbers, I would dread meeting them for a date in the daylight as they would be able to see me properly and I would be sober. These were the days of Blackberry Messenger, so I'd spend days and days BBMing some guys before it would all fall apart. I remember one guy asking me what I did and when I told him about the charity, he put two and two together and worked out who I was. He never contacted me again. He didn't even bother to make up a lame excuse, just ghosted me once he knew I had burns scars.

Another guy messaged me just before we were due to meet and asked if he could bring his auntie. I was totally thrown and asked why. 'She's a massive fan and she needs a job. I wondered if you had some work at your charity you could give her', he said. So much for it being a date.

Occasionally I'd make plans to meet up with someone for dinner and I'd go on recces to restaurants to check the lighting, trying to work out where would be the best place for me to sit so my injuries would be less visible. Even if I could get over the hurdle of the lighting, I also had a fear of eating in front of someone. My oesophagus had been stented, which means food can get trapped, causing me to choke. It was not ideal that I needed to either mash up my food like a small child or else face the possibility that my date would need to use the Heimlich manoeuvre on me.

Another time, I'd met my date when we'd both been drinking, so I couldn't tell whether he had clocked my injuries. He worked in the City (the financial district in London) and wanted to meet up for dinner. In spite of my fears, I agreed. We'd been messaging continually, plus speaking on the phone – chatting till we fell asleep at night – so it felt like we'd become close. I was skint at this point and he suggested a really nice restaurant, but I agreed to go because I thought there might be a possibility of this becoming a relationship. I definitely misjudged him.

As soon as he saw me, his face fell. It was obvious that he didn't know I had burns. He could barely make eye contact, his eyes darting round the restaurant, looking anywhere but at me. It was incredibly awkward, but we ordered. I tried to hide my shock when I saw on the menu that it was £15 for a cocktail, which I couldn't really afford. 'I've just seen some friends having dinner. I'll go and say "Hi" to them and be back in a minute', he said. And, guess what? He never came back. By the time the waiter had brought out all the food we'd ordered, it was obvious what had happened.

In my head, I tried to make up excuses for him, that maybe he'd had a panic attack or received an urgent phone call from work he had to deal with. But I knew the truth and I sat there with my bottom lip trembling, feeling utterly worthless and desperately trying to hold it together. To add insult to injury, I had to pay for everything and I couldn't even eat a mouthful of the stupidly expensive food, I was so upset.

The pattern continued, guy after guy doing the same thing – getting close on Messenger but then not being interested once we met up in person. Then, just before I went on a trip to the USA to film a documentary about stem cells, I met a guy who wanted to date me. A breakthrough! But, sadly, this had no Hollywood ending. He didn't seem to have any interest in working and lived in a filthy flat so, honestly, I don't know what I saw in him. Feeling sorry for him, I said he could use my flat while I was away. When I came back, I realised that not only had he brought girls back with him but he'd slept with them in my bed, and he walked off with a whole load of my stuff.

What a wake-up call. It made me take a long, hard look at the sorts of men I was pursuing. I have to be honest, I'd had awful partners before the attack, so there was no point in looking back with rose-tinted glasses and thinking that everything had been great then because it hadn't. I needed to stop going out with absolute losers who couldn't even get their act together. Why was I even interested in dating men who treated me so poorly? Was I willing to put up with all this just so I wouldn't be on my own? Was I that afraid of being single?

At this time, I was being interviewed regularly by journalists because of the documentary about me and subsequent TV work, and they often asked the same thing: 'Do you think you'll ever meet someone?' The question always came with a slightly sympathetic incline of the head, which made me feel pitied, so did nothing for my self-esteem. It always felt like people were invested, too, as though me meeting a romantic partner would mean there was a happy ending to my story. They could run the piece with a 'Poor Katie has been through so much but look at her now, happily in love' narrative. It felt so demeaning. Both the idea that I should be grateful for a man to even think about dating me, and the way to redeem my story – my life! – was to be in a romantic relationship.

I'm sure they meant the questions kindly – there was certainly no malice in them – but it continued to push the idea that marriage is the pinnacle, and I needed to find someone to share my life with if I wanted to be happy.

It's the story we've been hearing all our lives. We grew up watching Disney films where the princess always got her prince. They fell in love within seconds, often after he rescued her in some way, and then they lived happily ever after. As we got older, we moved on to romantic comedies like *Bridget Jones's Diary*, with Bridget being portrayed as a mess because she was a single woman, a size 12, and couldn't cook. But it was OK because Mark Darcy loved her.

So many of the TV programmes we watched and novels we read from our teenage years onwards have romantic themes. And you're far more likely to read a book in which someone looks for, or accidentally finds, their soulmate than one that focuses on friendships or careers. One study in 2018 estimated that, of all the top 40 songs between 1960 and 2010, 67.3 per cent were about love, and 29.9 per cent referenced sex.[1]

Over and over, we have been told in one way or another that romantic love is not only the most important part of our lives but also, finding it equals happiness. Men have often been painted as the saviours, meaning that red flags in romcoms can be ignored, so long as he has told the woman he loved her by the end (or, in the case of a certain popular steamy trilogy, he is super-rich). Romance is portrayed as consisting of longing glances and strong sexual attraction. Often we see them fall in love in a montage of happy clips with beautiful music playing over the top. We never hear what they talk about and very little emphasis is placed on what the couple has in common or what life looks like after they have declared their undying love for each other.

I'd like to think that society has changed since then and, to some extent, it has but, even more recently, an article appeared in *Newsweek* sharing the opinion that Taylor Swift is not a good role model for young girls: 'At 34, Swift remains unmarried and childless, a fact that some might argue is irrelevant to her status as a role model. But, I suggest, it's crucial to consider what kind of example this sets for young girls. A role model, by definition, is someone worthy of imitation. While Swift's musical talent and business acumen are certainly admirable, even laudable, we must ask if her personal life choices are ones we want our sisters and daughters to emulate.'[2] The patriarchy appears to be alive and kicking, berating one of the most creative, resilient, strong, courageous, and remarkable women of our generation for not being married and having babies by the age of 34. What a terrible example she is as she sells out world tours that bring happiness to millions, pausing only to donate to local foodbanks on her way.

The pressure we feel doesn't just come from the media, films, TV, and books; it can come at us from closer to home too. I know I'm not the only one to have been continually asked by friends and family whether I've met someone yet. I'd also heard many people refer to their spouse as their 'other half'. This seems like a harmless term, until you think through the implication, which is that we're not whole people if we are single.

When my earnings increased, I was able to do nice things but, if you go out for dinner, a table is never set for one, and you're likely to get a slightly pitying look from a waiter when you say it's just you. Buying food in the supermarket, things are rarely packaged for a single person. If you're looking to book a holiday, hotel rooms are far cheaper when there are two of you. There are tax breaks for married couples. It's much harder to get on the property ladder on one income. And so it goes on… Sometimes it feels like the world is set up for pairs.

Every time you fill in a form, you're asked to put yourself in a box based on whether you're married or not. So, for women, traditionally we've been forced to tell the world whether we're Miss or Mrs, while men remain Mr regardless because their marital status hasn't ever mattered in the same way that ours does. That said, I'm sure many men face pressure from society and loved ones to be in a relationship but, if they're single, they get to be the sexy bachelor while we get stuck with being the old maid or spinster who is 'on the shelf'. A single man with a dog? Cute! Single woman with a cat? Crazy cat lady!

While women tend to get married later than they did 50 years ago,[3] society is still more geared up to celebrate marriage and motherhood than singleness. Strangely, this seems to increase with each generation. Proposals are sometimes much more public events than they were, with some people arranging for a photographer to hide somewhere nearby to capture the magical moment when they pop the question. Baby showers, an American celebration, were coming into fashion in the UK at the start of the new millennium, but now gender reveal parties have been added. There are engagement parties and huge weddings, with so much pressure to get every detail Instagrammably perfect.

Engagements, marriages, and births are wonderful events to celebrate, but how much attention do we pay to other events in women's lives? How many graduation parties have you been to? When you or a friend gets a promotion or is starting an exciting new job, how much do you celebrate together? Have you ever taken a friend out to dinner to celebrate how long you've been in each other's lives? Where are the greetings cards that say, 'Well done for getting out of a crap relationship!', 'You hit your running goal – congratulations!', or 'You're amazing – you keep going to therapy and dealing with your childhood trauma!' We don't celebrate many achievements like these in our lives, so it can feel like everything points towards finding your one true love.

If it feels like our lives are building towards the crescendo of falling in love, getting married, and having children, it's no wonder that looking at our later 40s and beyond can feel like falling off a cliff for many of us. It's been built up and built up that this is the purpose of our life, the zenith of all our hopes and dreams. But then what? If it doesn't happen for us, what then? If it does, but we then end up divorced, what then? If we stay married and realise that reality is not like the fantasy, it takes a lot of hard work, what does that mean? If we become mothers and find it challenging and exhausting rather than something that continually fulfils and delights us, have we done something wrong? When our kids need us less or leave home, are we washed up and useless?

The truth is that life is not a fairy tale and romance does not overcome every one of our problems. If it did, all married people would be on cloud nine all the time. The idea that true love and happiness awaits us in one other human being is a fantasy. Hear me right: I'm not knocking love, romance, and relationships. Of course there can be a huge amount of joy in finding someone you want to spend your life with. But that is not our sole purpose for being. If we place our happiness in the hands of one person, it's a recipe for disaster. No relationship should have that much pressure put on it. No one can make us feel completely fulfilled for ever more. All human beings are just that – human – so are fallible and flawed. No one is perfect and, however much we

The truth is that life is not a fairy tale and romance doesn't answer every one of our problems.

love someone, we still let them down and disappoint them at times, and they will do the same to us. That's simply the way it is.

The myth is that being in a romantic relationship will mean an end to loneliness, but loneliness isn't simply about being on your own. You can feel far lonelier in a relationship when you aren't connecting with your partner than if you're contentedly on your own. Even if you're happy in your relationship, you can still feel lonely because, again, one person can't fill all our emotional needs.

I found it really interesting that actor and activist Rose McGowan pointed out in her book *Brave* that, 'We need to look at why so many women believe a man is going to save us. It's not because of any evidence of saving... It's just male-dominated society that snows us into not noticing it's we women doing the saving. We are the white stallion and we have to wait for no one but ourselves.'[4] It got me thinking about the evidence around me and I realised how often it is that it's women who do the saving, the patching up, the sorting out. Women so often take care of the children as well as elderly relatives, make the trips to the care homes, check in on members of the extended family. It can be so easy to look to a guy to be the saviour and then, years down the line, realise that you're the one doing all the saving.

The huge emphasis placed on finding a romantic partner can affect other parts of our life. With such a focus on sexual relationships, we can end up giving very little thought to finding, building, and maintaining friendships, and this can be detrimental. As Zara Abrams says in an article in the American Psychological Association's magazine *Monitor on Psychology*, 'Psychological research from around the world shows that having social connections is one of the most reliable predictors of a long, healthy, and satisfying life' and friendships 'can protect against mental health issues such as depression and anxiety.'[5] So why do we push them to the side, like they're not as important as a romantic partner? There are so many self-help books on how to find, improve, or restore a romantic relationship, but if you want to find out more about navigating different elements of friendship, there are only slim pickings.

Talk of friendships can bring up insecurities. While the majority of Western society ascribes to us having a romantic relationship with just one person, you can – in theory – have as many friends as you want. But this can lead to a fear and us asking, 'Do I have enough friends?' Emotionally, we can find ourselves back in the school playground, desperately wanting to be the most popular kid in class. For me, one of the joys of getting older has been realising that it's not about the quantity of friendships, it's about how deep they are. No one can sustain a large number of truly deep relationships, but if you've got one or two people you can count on, that will make all the difference.

What if we've lost friendships over the years and are feeling a bit lonely? Political activist, actress, and icon, Jane Fonda, who is in her mid-80s, is a huge advocate of cultivating female friendships and says, 'You have to be intentional… I never used to be intentional… You have to pursue people that you want to be friends with… and you have to say, "I'm intentionally wanting to be your friend."'[6] And it works. People hear that and then they stick around, and you develop new friendships.' Fellow actress Sally Field said Fonda knocked on her door and said, 'Come on, we're going to lunch.'[7] They've been close friends for about 40 years.

Friendship was different when we were younger. When we were in school, we were automatically around people the same age as us for much of the day, so friendships sprang out of those times relatively easily. Some are lucky enough to have work colleagues they connect and form good friendships with, but the move towards working from home can make that harder. The solution is to actively pursue people we think we could develop a good friendship with, like Fonda says. Thinking of it a bit more like dating and making an effort with the people we connect with, intentionally spending time together and investing in the relationship rather than simply hoping a good friendship will land in our lap, can really help.

Friendship can be such a gift to us at any stage of life. I'd pictured buying my first home with a partner and moving in together, so when it was my parents who dropped me off at my new flat when I moved back to London, I felt a bit deflated. As they headed home, I looked around at all the flat-pack furniture I'd bought and tried to summon up the energy to build it. 'Come on!' I thought, 'I don't need a man, I can do this!' But I couldn't even understand the first instruction. After a few minutes of fantasising about a wonderful, handsome man 'rescuing' me, I texted some mates. They rallied round, showing up at different times during the next couple of weeks. They brought wine and we'd open it as we started building the furniture and unpacking boxes. The alcohol definitely led to some wonky Billy bookcases, but they made me smile every time I saw them, reminding me how much we'd laughed while we were putting them together. When I let go of the fantasy of a handyman boyfriend (who, of course, I would never argue with over how to build furniture, so total fantasy), I realised that my reality was already pretty brilliant.

Likewise, when I wanted to go to New York, I would happily have taken a partner with me but, without one on the scene, I didn't need to miss out on having company, so I took my sister.

We timed it so we were there around her birthday. I snuck some balloons and banners into my suitcase and, while she was asleep, I decorated our hotel room, so she woke up to a birthday surprise. I booked a place that I'd heard was great for breakfast and asked them to put a candle in her waffle. These were the sorts of things I'd previously reserved for doing in romantic relationships but, doing them for my sister, I realised that I wanted to put the same level of effort and energy I'd invest in a man into investing in my family and friends, not less. They are going to be around for the long haul and those relationships are to be treasured. It was a liberating trip and we still talk about how much fun we had all these years later.

The less focus we put on friendships, the more pressure we put on romantic relationships to be our everything. The more pressure we put on marriage as the be-all and end-all of life, the less likely it is to live up to that. One person can't be our world, no matter how good that sounds on social media.

Friendship expert and motivational speaker Marisa G. Franco argues that friendships can actually enhance our romantic relationships and help us to cope better with any difficulties in that relationship. She says, 'if we are investing all of our resources in one person, when that relationship is not going well, it's going to affect us all the more, in ways that don't allow us to be grounded and return to a relationship in ways that can improve it, save it, rescue it'. She also says that she encourages those in a romantic relationship to maintain other friendships, as, 'our wellbeing is greater when we have what's called emotionships, which are different people that we can turn to to deal with different types of emotions'. This can be good for our partner as well as us because, she continues, 'Research also finds that when we connect with people outside of our marriage, not only do we become less depressed but our positive mood spills over to our partners so they become slightly less depressed as well.'

Not only are our friendships good for us when we're single, they're good for us full stop. We don't have friends as a consolation prize until we get married; they can bring so much to our lives no matter what else is happening.

In my own case, I grew up believing that my main goal should be to meet a man and he would look after me. Of course, that illusion was completely shattered when I later came to such harm at the hands of men but, up until then, there was another aspect of this belief. Although my parents told me I should work hard and earn my own money, I'd imbibed society's unwritten rule that the man should be the 'provider' in a relationship. I knew that women usually earned far less than men, so it seemed logical that if I wanted to have children, I would need someone who could take care of us financially. It felt as though society was built on women needing to be dependent on men (though I also saw the complete double standard applied to women as then they would be called gold-diggers).

Living in London, without a man on the scene, I was starting to earn my own money and, for the first time, knew that I would be able to provide for myself. I was also starting to realise that, before I could get into a healthy relationship, I had to change the mindset I'd accepted for so long and fully embrace the fact that I didn't *need* a man to be happy. I wanted to be sure that if I were to be in a relationship, it would be because it was good for me, not just to conform to society's expectations of women. I couldn't put my happiness into the hands of someone else just to be provided for, and I was willing to work hard to do this for myself, to create the life I wanted and I could be proud of.

My next move was to enrol on an acting course. Not because

I wanted to be an actress, but because I knew it would bolster my confidence when meeting new people. I'd started being invited to work events and now I didn't let the fact that I didn't have a plus one stop me from going. Before, I'd feared that I would feel pathetic on my own but, actually, it meant I spoke to lots of interesting people and there was no worrying about whether my plus one was having a good time. I also took the initiative and invited friends and new acquaintances out for drinks. I tried new restaurants on my own and smiled confidently as I asked for a table for one. I got into fitness, finding a personal trainer to help me build up my strength. I started looking at what the options were for me to have children, investigating adoption, sperm donation, and freezing my eggs for the future.

Taking control helped to a certain extent, but didn't completely take away the desire to meet someone and I wouldn't want to pretend that it did. Sometimes the narrative around singleness swings from a patronising, 'Oh, poor you, it's so sad you're alone', to a militant cry like, 'A woman needs a man like a fish needs a bicycle!' Neither extreme is particularly helpful. It's natural to want to be in a relationship and if you're single and you'd rather not be, I hope you find someone. I also hope that if you don't or you're in a relationship that comes to an end, you know that you've still got plenty of good things in your life. For me, making some positive decisions about how I spend my time and focusing on what I had rather than what I didn't have helped me to gain confidence and see what a full life I could lead, whether I met someone or not.

Ultimately, we are the heroes of our own stories. We're not the Disney princesses of old, waiting to be rescued. I love Cher's attitude to this. She'd been quoted as saying, 'A man is not a necessity, a man is a luxury.' When asked about this, she added,

'My mom said to me, "You know, sweetheart, one day you should settle down and marry a rich man." And I said, "Mom, I *am* a rich man."'[9]

When we are our own hero, we don't have to wait around for one to fly in to save us. There is so much more to living our life. It isn't a matter of choosing either romance, marriage, and motherhood or career and friendship. Nor is it about elevating one or the other. The fact is that *all* these things are valid. They can all be expressions of who you are and the ways you want to show up in the world.

Once you've got married and had children, there's then a lot of pressure to be fulfilled by being a wife and mother, a lot of expectation for these roles to be our everything, but it's OK to find it hard. Presumably that's why so many romantic films finish at the point when the couple get together, because what comes next can be mundane and hard work.

Living with another person is difficult. We're by nature selfish creatures (who wouldn't want things the way they want them?!), so having to adjust to take into account someone else's desires requires ongoing compromise from both parties. Relationships take work. We need to know this deep down or we'll forever be disappointed, wondering if there's someone better for us somewhere.

The truth is, every relationship has its highs and lows. We can't judge our own marriage by what we perceive other people's to be like. The phrase, 'You never know what is going on behind closed doors' is entirely true. You can't compare the day-to-day realities of your relationship or the fact it's going through a hard patch to what you see in the life of someone else who's in their honeymoon period and is only sharing their highlights on social media.

Finding friends we can be real with about our romantic

relationships can really help, like a safety valve, allowing some of the pressure to escape and enabling us to decipher whether we've had a row simply because we're exhausted or there's something more serious that we need to look into. It's also such a relief when you can vocalise something you're struggling with and a friend says that they've been there and they know what it's like.

After a couple of years being single, a friend introduced me to Richie. We were just friends at first but, when I was away filming in America for a few weeks, we started messaging more and speaking on the phone regularly. We became close, but lived a couple of hours away from each other, so one of us would have to make the long journey on a Friday night after work to enable us to spend the weekend together.

Not long after we became romantically involved, I got an infection in my nose that meant I needed another operation. My instinct was I should let Richie off the hook – it didn't seem fair for him to take on all my medical needs when we'd only been dating for a short time. But he wouldn't have any of it. 'We get on so well,' he said, 'why give up now?' I thought he was being sweet but naive. 'As soon as he sees me in hospital', I thought, 'bedridden, with a splint on my face, and a drain to remove the fluid and puss from the wound, he'll run for the hills.' Instead, when he turned up after the operation with Hula Hoops, the latest *Grazia* magazine, and a packet of wine gums, he settled down to chat and seemed completely relaxed about the whole thing.

When I left hospital, I thought he would be embarrassed to be seen with me, with my walking stick and my nose all swollen and black while it healed, but he insisted I accompany him on our usual trip to Blockbuster to pick up a couple of DVDs and some popcorn for our night in. His kindness and lack of concern about what I looked like was a world away from the men I'd dated before who'd treated me so badly.

Don't let this fool you into thinking that we then just rode off into the sunset to live happily ever after. Our relationship, like any relationship, has had its challenges. There's been a lot to think about and navigate over the years, not least of which was what to do when we had kids. We knew that one of us would let their career take a back seat so our children could be well cared for. I took maternity leave to be with both our daughters, and there have been periods when work has been quieter for me, so I was around more then. However, as my career took off, often it was Richie who was picking things up at home. That all took some working through.

When we met, I was far less confident and outgoing than I am now, so I've changed a lot. That, in turn, altered the dynamics of our relationship and how it works. At various points, my health challenges have turned our lives upside down, sometimes with very little warning. Life doesn't stay the same, so we've had to work hard at sustaining our relationship throughout. There have been times when we've not been able to see a way forward and considered splitting up. It's come so close that Richie even moved out for a while as we both needed some space. We kept it really private and didn't even tell our families. Thankfully, we were able to find a way through it and stay together.

I say all this so that you don't see pictures of us on Instagram and think that we have a perfect relationship. We love each other, and the photos and videos of us having fun and enjoying each other's company are all real, but they're not the whole picture. Social media is only ever a glimpse. There is no one perfect person for us, someone who will never wind us up or let us down, and there is no such thing as a perfect relationship where no one makes mistakes. That said, for all its ups and downs, I love being married, and I've found it's got better as we've got older.

I also love being a mum to our two girls, but being married and having kids doesn't mean that I love the other aspects of my life any less. I still put a lot of time and energy into my voluntary and paid work. I still prioritise exercise and looking after my body. I still enjoy spending time with other members of the family and friends.

There can be real pressure to put our kids first 24/7 and put the rest of your life on hold until they've grown up, but I don't think that serves either them or us well. We are not machines that can give out endlessly. Yes, a huge part of being a parent *is* giving sacrificially to our kids, but we also need to find ways to recharge and explore other aspects of who we are. Just in case you need to hear this, it doesn't make us bad people if we enjoy spending time at work, going to the gym, or meeting up with friends. It probably makes us more rounded individuals and better examples for our kids.

It's very hard for us women to say that our needs matter (we'll look at this in more detail in Chapter 9), but this is especially true when we talk about us as mothers. There's such a fear that if we say we want or need to do something that's about us as individuals, people will think we don't love our kids or we're not taking proper care of them. Women get shamed for wanting to do things outside the family, whereas it's not only absolutely fine, but actually *expected*, for men to do so. Society still hasn't got used to the idea of men wanting to stay at home with their kids or spend more time with them, so we think nothing of them travelling for work or prioritising their achievements. We don't even expect them to talk about whether they're a father or not, let alone define themselves as such.

I firmly believe we shouldn't be ashamed to say that we don't get all our fulfilment from one person or one role in our lives. Despite what the majority of all those romcoms taught us, romance isn't what we need, connection is. Connection with ourselves, connection with different people, and different activities that tap into different parts of us and make us feel alive in a variety of ways. No one person can be everything to us, and no one role in life can fulfil us completely. This is brilliant news for when we look ahead to the rest of our lives!

We don't build up to a peak of being newly-weds and having newborns and that's it. Those days can be amazing (and exhausting, confusing, disappointing, difficult), but there are other fantastic things to come. It's not a case of the best life has to offer is now in the past and it's all downhill from here – there is so much more ahead! More that will bring us joy, new and changing roles to stretch and shape us in different ways. There may be things to come that we've been wondering about for years but haven't had the time to act on with a young family or a burgeoning career. Maybe there's a charity or a local cause that you'd love to volunteer for, a hobby you'd like to pursue but just haven't had the time to really invest in it. For many of us there comes a time in our lives when we realise that we've not seen our friends as much as we would have liked in recent years. It can be surprisingly easy, though, to reconnect and rekindle old relationships, and find joy in what they bring out in us.

Life is continually shifting, pulling us in different directions. When we lose something, it makes space for something else. If we have kids, our relationship with them will change naturally as they grow up. Mine are still young, so I haven't yet got to the point where they are out more than they're home, but I know that day

I firmly believe we shouldn't be ashamed to say that we don't get all our fulfilment from one person or one role in our lives.

will come and, just as it did when they were born, my life will shift again, making more space for other things. I will continue to pour myself into motherhood and prioritise the wellbeing of my girls, but I will hold on to the fact that I have other things to bring to the world too.

When I watch Disney films with my girls, I see that the messages they convey are changing. Little girls now are enthralled by Elsa's powers rather than just her pretty dresses. *Frozen* has also taught them that an act of true love can come from someone other than a man, and the importance of sisterhood. That's progress. Similarly, Moana doesn't need a man to save the day and, in fact, her male sidekick is more of a hindrance than a hero. *Encanto* focuses on the importance of family and that we are all worthy of love.

Modern female Disney characters, then, spend less time waiting to be rescued and more time making things happen, pushing against the expectations placed on them by others, finding ways to be strong and brave, and writing their own stories. Now, if they could include even more diverse characters, show the reality of what happens in long-term relationships, acknowledge that divorce exists, and start writing stories about older women, well, society will have truly changed.

Until then, let's keep writing and validating our own stories, whatever they may be. Let's set our own standards for how we want our lives to look, and not be defined by society's expectations of women. Let's embrace the changing seasons of life, not fear them, knowing that every time one of our roles in life shifts, it makes space for new things. Remember, connections come in all sorts of shapes and sizes and each one brings something to our lives. Let's look ahead to the future, rejecting the premise that we are defined by our marital status or motherhood, and knowing that we are so much more – and there is so much more to come.

A moment to pause
•••

What does it mean for you to be the hero of your own story? What do you want for yourself as you see what, historically, society's expectations have been in the past of what women should want and do?

7

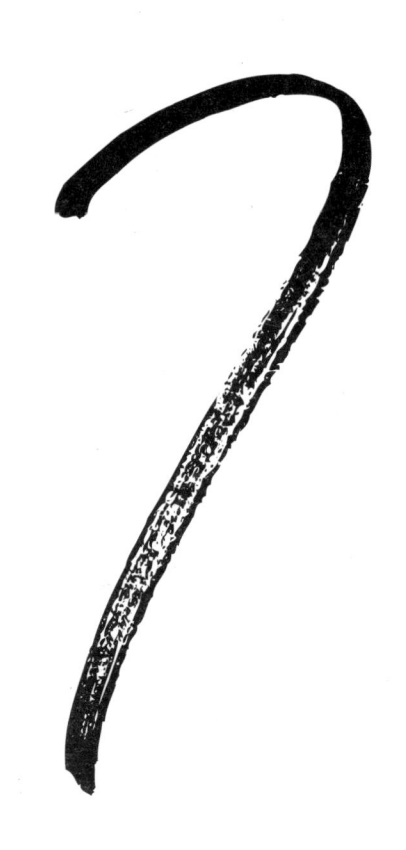

Old is not a dirty word

There have been four times in my life when I thought I was going to die. In the hotel room where I was raped in 2008, when I was attacked with acid on the street days later, when I had surgical emphysema at the end of 2008, and when I had sepsis in 2019. Each time, there was a very real possibility that my life would end. I had also felt suicidal when I was in hospital recovering from the acid attack, unable to see a reason to keep living, and so was working out the best way to take my life.

The stark reality of these events in my past meant that it really confused me when people started asking, with a slight grimace and sympathetic tilt of the head, how I felt about turning 40. How did I feel? Ecstatic! I never thought I would make it, and there were certainly times when I couldn't have imagined that I'd be enjoying my life even if I had. Seeing 40 on the horizon wasn't something I feared; it was something I relished. It was close, so I might make it after all! I wasn't going to hide away from it and pretend it wasn't happening, I was happy about it and planned on throwing a party and inviting all my friends and family to celebrate with me.

I'd also been following closely the journey of Deborah James, who became known as Bowelbabe after she was diagnosed with bowel cancer at the age of 35 and worked to raise awareness of the disease. She recorded a podcast called You, Me and the Big C

How could I possibly even think of moaning about my age when Deborah would have loved to have carried on living and, therefore, had the opportunity to be ageing like me?

in which she talked about her life with cancer with humour and honesty. In some ways, she reminded me of myself. We were the same age, both had young families, both loved make-up and sequins, and would get dressed up for our hospital appointments. Her mum even looked like my mum and would go to every hospital appointment with her, just as my mum did for me. Like many others, I fell in love with Deborah's indomitable spirit and was incredibly sad when she passed away. She died when she was 40, so she came to mind whenever someone would ask me if I was daunted about entering a new decade. What happened to her brought things into sharp focus for me. How could I possibly even think of moaning about my age when Deborah would have loved to have carried on living and, therefore, had the opportunity to be ageing like me?

The negative questions and thoughts about my reaching this age got me asking questions too. Are we all looking back at our youth through rose-tinted glasses? We can romanticise our youth, remembering long, hot summers, the joy of first love, the fun we had with our mates. We can also forget about the frustrations of being that age – the lack of true autonomy, arguments with our friends, insecurities around our crushes, and the looming question, 'What do you want to do with the rest of your life?'

When we were children, we had virtually no control over our lives and our happiness was dependent on things like whether we had loving and stable caregivers, how we fitted into the school system, and how good our teachers were. Even if we are lucky enough to have loving parents, they are still subject to things outside their control: illness, accidents, money problems, addictions, relationship breakdown. I don't need to tell you that school can be hard. The education system scores us, deciding whether we pass or fail. We don't have the luxury of opting out of subjects that we're not suited to until we're towards the end of our education. We're continually assessed, judged, reported on, told what to do, how to behave, when we can have a break, and when and how hard we have to work.

Of course, most parents and teachers want us to do the best we can at school because doing well can open up the maximum number of doors for us. Often, it's only as we get older that we realise the system doesn't work for everyone and there are alternatives. We hear about entrepreneurs who failed all their exams, yet went on to have remarkably successful careers. We also see friends who did well academically make some really bad choices in life. Some of us go through our adult lives thinking that we're stupid because we didn't fit into any of the boxes school wanted us to.

If you do well at school academically, that doesn't necessarily mean you'll do well socially, which is another huge aspect of our life when we're young. There's massive pressure to fit in, be like everyone else, and do the things they're doing. We're not cookie cutter people so of course we're not all the same, interested in the same things, wanting to wear the same clothes, and so on, but we can fear that if we step out of line, we'll become the butt of some joke because we're different. At such a young age, we don't know what will be important to us 20 years down the line. We make short-term decisions, many of them unwise, because we don't know any better. Our sense of self is malleable and we find our identity shifting with different friendship groups, relationships, and trends. We give everyone else the power to judge us, but don't give our own judgements the same level of credence.

When we move on to our 20s, we're still dealing with many of the same insecurities as before, but also trying to work out what job we want to do and how to get it. At the same time, we're likely to be navigating big changes like leaving home, finding rented accommodation, living with flatmates, and becoming responsible for bills and the domestic chores. We're falling in and out of love, with all the highs and lows that entails as we learn how to have adult relationships, or else desperately wanting to be in the perfect romantic relationship, but having to work out what single life looks like in a world obsessed with finding 'the one'.

Then there's the pressure of our 30s. If we haven't hit certain milestones – relationship, engagement, marriage, kids – we feel like we're on a game show with a giant clock counting down and reminding us that time is running out and we're missing the targets society says define us. If we become mothers, we're expected to put the rest of our life on hold and give our children everything, otherwise we're not considered good mums (meanwhile, men are congratulated for looking after their own children for a day and hailed as heroes for being 'hands-on dads'). All this against a background of trying to establish and progress our career in a world that is still heavily misogynistic, or pausing it to meet our family commitments, then wondering what this means for our future.

So, after all this navigating, after all the challenges we've faced and overcome so far (many more as well that we've not been able to cover in these few paragraphs), are we really supposed to think that life is over at 40? That was it?! The truth is, if our life expectancy is 83,[1] then we've still got a lot of living to do! We're only halfway there and, as anyone who has ever taken on a running challenge knows, the halfway point never feels anywhere near the end. It seems to me that we've done an awful lot of learning in our first 40 years. Chances are that we've made a lot of mistakes in this time as we've tried to work out who we are and what we want our lives to look like, which means we've likely learned a lot too. We've been building some solid foundations for making the most of the second 40 years.

As well as just being thankful to be alive, I was thankful for the ways I've changed over the years. I look back at my 21-year-old self and I see now that I was a screaming bag of insecurities. There wasn't a scratch on my body, not a hair out of place, yet I wasn't truly comfortable in my own skin. I thought I was – after all, I was posing for lads' mags in tiny bikinis. I thought I oozed confidence, but I was desperate for approval and attention. I had no self-belief and needed other people to tell me I was beautiful, glamorous, sexy, worthy of love. I sought affection and affirmation in all the wrong places. My body may have been considered damn near perfect by the fashion industry, but my self-confidence was on the floor.

Now, despite all that's happened, I love my body, with all her foibles and flaws, because she's mine and she's amazing. I'm not going to pretend that I never look at other women and feel envious of their bodies or feel less than them because of mine, but I try to let those feelings go as quickly as they came. I don't let them hang around for as long as I did when I was younger. We all have moments of self-doubt and feeling inadequate, but I try to remember that someone else is trying to profit from me feeling like that so I don't feed it. I'm not here to compete with anyone and no one wins at the game of comparison.

I am no longer desperate to fit in and be like everyone else like I was at school. I don't let other people's judgements take precedence over my own judgements any more. My opinion not only counts, it outweighs the opinions of anyone else who wants to judge me. They don't know me, they don't live in my skin and

Once I let go of the stigma that is attached to ageing and started looking around me at what older women are really like, I was amazed, encouraged, and inspired.

know what it's like to have my heart, or my thoughts, so why would I let them dictate how I should live? I've also realised that people are probably judging me a lot less than I think they are. Most of them probably don't give me a second thought.

I judge myself differently too. I used to feel so bad every time I made a mistake, but now I try to make sure my inner voice is kind and that I use the tone and words I would if I were speaking to a friend in that situation. If I get turned down for something – a work thing I'd been hoping to do, say – I don't assume that's happened because I'm no good. I just think that it wasn't meant for me but something else will be.

Once I let go of the stigma that is attached to ageing and started looking around me at what older women are really like, I was amazed, encouraged, and inspired. Among family, friends, and work colleagues I saw that, compared with younger women, they have greater self-awareness – they know who they are and what they want. They are more comfortable with setting boundaries and saying no. They are less interested in trying to align with society's expectations and content to just be themselves.

This helped me to see that I don't need to be perfect to be happy with who I am. I love how actor Hannah Waddingham put it, 'You get to an age, for me in my late 40s, where you're done with trying to perfect yourself. When you're OK with the fact you've got jagged edges and delicious spikey bits that don't want to be moulded into something. It's very nice to feel like that.'[2] Doesn't that make you want to exhale? It's wonderfully freeing realising that you're at a life stage when you can let go, stop carrying everyone else's expectations and judgements around with you, and make peace with yourself.

I love hearing women talking, too, about how they've learned to trust themselves over time. Author Glennon Doyle calls it deep self-care. She posted a video explaining what deep self-care – true self-care – is and this quote from her book *Untamed*: "'I love myself now. Self-love means that I have a relationship with myself built on trust and loyalty. I trust myself to have my own back, so my allegiance is to the voice within. I'll abandon everyone else's expectations of me before I'll abandon myself. I'll disappoint everyone else before I'll disappoint myself. I'll forsake all others before I'll forsake myself. Me and myself: We are till death do us part. What the world needs is more women who have quit fearing themselves and starting trusting themselves." *Untamed*.[3]

What a rallying cry! We all hope that there will be people who'll be by our side at different stages of our lives, but the only person we can guarantee will be there from the first to the last day is us! This is why we need to root for ourselves, to be our own biggest cheerleader and biggest defender. We have to trust that our intuition, our gut, is for us and trying to look out for us. I used to ignore that little voice inside. Sometimes I couldn't even hear her over the noise of other people's opinions. But now I know, from years of experience, that my intuition can be relied on to tell me what work projects will bring me the most fulfilment, who I'm likely to become friends with in a group of people, who I will work well alongside, who I should avoid, and what activities I should spend my time on. If you're not convinced that this knowing can be a superpower, a government report in 2015 encouraged the intelligence services in the UK to employ more middle-aged women for their high levels of emotional intelligence and intuition gained from their 'valuable life experience'.[4] Midlife isn't the beginning of the end; we're coming into our own.

This inner knowing – a confidence in ourselves and our abilities to make good choices – gives us the courage to act. One of the benefits of being older is that we've got so much more

Midlife isn't the beginning of the end; we're coming into our own.

experience. When we tried something new at 21, we didn't know how it would work out, so could be paralysed by fear or gutted if it didn't turn out as expected. Now we know two things: we can do more than perhaps we thought possible; if we can't do something, we will survive. Failure isn't final and consistency counts for more than we give it credit for. We get better at everything if we keep going. Think of all the things we've spent hundreds, if not thousands, of hours doing so far in our lives. When starting out in a new career, we can feel daunted, but when we've racked up 10 or 20 years' experience, we know what we're doing, whether we give ourselves credit for it or not. Being around other people who draw out the best in us can also add to our confidence over the years, as it shows us that others believe in us, even when we don't believe in ourselves.

When I'm in a board meeting and need some advice, I look to the people who have the relevant life experience to be able to help. Sometimes these will be younger people who've been through a lot, which has led to them gaining maturity and wisdom at an early age, but often they'll be the older people in the group. That's because I need to hear from those who have been there before, who have the insight and knowledge we need in that moment. Sometimes I'll specifically seek out women in TV who have earned their stripes. I know that I'll be able to learn a lot from them because they've seen it all and survived to tell the tale. This is the case even when they've made mistakes on the way – it only serves to make what they have to say more valuable. Disastrous experiences not only make for great stories, they teach us so much. There's a wisdom and gravitas that only comes with age.

When I meet a woman who's over 40, I know she'll have a story or two to tell – difficulties she's overcome, lessons she's learned. We don't pick up nearly so much from people who make out like they've always had their lives together, which is why I'd much rather hear from people who have walked through fire and come out the other side. I find people's life experiences so interesting, and when I see other women flourishing despite having made mistakes, it helps me to worry less about my own. Mistakes are part of a life well lived!

One of the things I admire most in older women is the fact that so many stop taking any crap and I think I know why this is. I've noticed that the more I know what I want, the more the weight of other people's judgements lifts, leaving me free to stand up for myself. I only see that increasing as I get older.

I saw a fascinating interview with screen legend Sharon Stone on how she felt at 60.[5] She said that people think no one fancies you any more, but she's found that just as many men want to sleep with her as they ever did. The difference, she reasoned, is that men know women aren't 'as easy' when they're older. They are still hot, but not as easy to get rid of, to put up with being a bit on the side, or to keep quiet. The older we get, the more we know what we want and it's not to be treated badly! We're done with the patriarchal bullshit! Female friends who are dating men at my age and older say that they've noticed this too. The more content they become with themselves, the less they feel like they need a man or are willing to put up with things. They have no interest in jumping through hoops to prove themselves worthy of love, and they can spot the decent men much faster than when they were younger.

The more we stand up for ourselves and find our voice, the more likely it is that some people – some men especially – may see us as 'difficult'. That can be a hard label for us to deal with because, since we were little girls, we've been trained to make life easier for other people and not to 'cause a fuss'. So when someone calls us difficult, what they really mean is that we're no longer pliable, we're happy to put ourselves first, and unwilling to accept the scraps of someone's time and attention because we know our own worth. If men can feed us the narrative that we should be grateful for them to even look our way, they can keep us accepting less than what we're worth. But men who dismiss the idea of dating older women only short-change themselves because, again, our worth is not in our youth. The older we get, the more we bring to the table, and it saddens me to see older men choosing far younger women as they're missing out on strong, resilient, confident, capable women their own age. Although, perhaps those women have had a lucky escape.

In a related way, I've felt that my face has become an idiot filter. It causes some people to reject me immediately and I'm OK with that as it helps me to avoid the people I don't want in my life. People who judge others so superficially or on aesthetics are not for me. Some heterosexual women say ageing is like that: if a man rejects you because of your age, he's not worthy of you. Better, too, that he rejects you early on and shows his true colours than you invest heavily in the relationship and only find out how shallow he is further down the line.

From my own experience, I think that, as we get older, we learn how to accept love differently too. I look back and see that my insecurities as a young person made me quite toxic. I would reject stable, kind, and considerate men because I thought they were boring. I interpreted jealousy as meaning that a man really liked me, and a chaotic life as an interesting one. As I got older, more secure and calm, and understood myself better, I was able to accept the love of a kind and decent man, realising that it was exactly what I needed. There was no need to play games with each other, pretending we weren't interested when we were. I was no longer looking for dangerous excitement; I wanted someone who would love me in the way that I deserved. It took ageing for me to be ready to receive good things.

The older we get, the more we also seem to understand that we need to look after and advocate for ourselves. There will be people in our lives who will try to take care of us, but you're the only one living in your body so you're the only one who knows what you really need. We'll talk a bit more about true self-care (not the bubble bath and candle kind we've been sold) in Chapter 9, but I just want to mention here that I have learned a lot from writer Kathy Lette, author of 20 books. She says, 'Once you're through the menopause, your oestrogen levels drop, which is your caring, sharing hormone, and your testosterone comes up. So for the first time ever, you get a little bit more bolshie, a little bit more selfish – a little bit more like a bloke, actually – and you put yourself first. I would say to women: "You've put yourself second your whole life; this is the time for you. So carpe the hell out of diem."'[6]

Kathy was 65 when we met and she was fabulous, funny, fierce, and full of life, with far more energy and sex appeal than most 20-year-olds. She talked about a concept she calls 'the second act', explaining that the menopause is like the interval in the performance of a play, and if we can just get through the interval, then we can enjoy the second act – the other half of our life – to the full. She described our childhood, teens, and 20s as being the 'hard life' and how, in our 40s, we begin to enter the 'soft life'.

I could really relate. It feels like there's so much pressure in our 20s and 30s – everyone is telling us that we need to find a good man, a good career, start having a family. It can feel competitive, even brutal at times, and mean that you have to harden yourself to get through it. In our 40s we can feel less desperate to keep moving forward so it's softer. We've worked through some of the messages society keeps impressing on us and realised that, actually, we don't need to do or have everything that we're told to live a contented life. Once we are less concerned with the judgements and criticisms of others, we're more confident and feel happier and sexier than ever before, ready for adventure.

So no, we don't need to view big birthdays and the ageing process as a dirty secret, something we should be ashamed of and hide at all costs. Increasingly, women are taking to social media and laying claim to their years with an honesty that wasn't seen even a decade ago. They have realised that there's not only nothing to be ashamed of but also their years have bought them the clout they didn't have when they were younger. We need to keep challenging the ageism we've internalised and start to see some of the many benefits of ageing. There are so many things we can bring to society at this stage in our life that we couldn't have hoped to when we were 20 or even 30. I'm not saying that we hit 40 and, suddenly, we don't have any worries. We've been fighting some of our battles since we were little girls trying to find our place in the world and there's no magic bullet that will make them disappear. But I think that we do find respite from them and begin to understand more about what we want and need to have a life we're proud of.

We can take inspiration from the women who've come before us, the ones who took risks and learned lessons that we can benefit from. We can hold on to the wisdom people like Deborah James shared with us – that life is a gift and we shouldn't take it for granted because we never know how long we've got. She

Let's not wait until we're staring death in the face before we start to enjoy life.

urged us to have as much fun as possible and said that her cancer diagnosis gave her an appreciation for things in her life that she'd never had before.[7]

Let's not wait until we're staring death in the face before we start to enjoy life. We don't have to buy into the idea that it's all downhill after 40 and we've got nothing to offer society. We don't need to play it safe, live as though we're just waiting for our life to end with our best days behind us. We can grab life with both hands and wring every drop of experience from it. Rather than staying at home, moaning about our sagging body, we can take that sagging body down to the beach and jump into the sea. We can worry about being rejected or making a mistake or we can put ourselves out there and really live, knowing that the worst-case scenario is we'll learn a lesson and have a good story to tell our friends if it goes wrong. The past has gone. The future is unknown, but what we do have is right now, so let's make the most of it. Maybe life is just getting started.

A moment to pause
•••

As you look at who you are now, compared with who you were in your 20s, what do you most want to celebrate? As you think about some of the benefits of continuing to age, what quality would you most like
to possess?

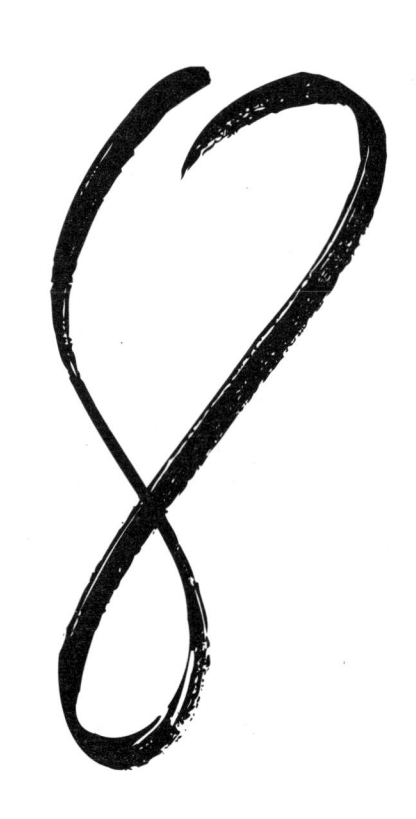

A change of perspective

I was sitting in a plush chair in a beautiful hotel in the centre of London, looking out at the incredible views of the city. Believe me when I say that this isn't what a normal day looks like for me. Behind me hung an exquisite floor-length gown (so different from the gym gear that I spend half my life in) and, on the desk beside me, nestled in its box, waiting to be worn, was a stunning ruby necklace loaned to me by Fabergé. Next to it lay a thick, embossed card. It was my invitation to that evening's British Academy Film and Television Arts (BAFTA) Awards ceremony.

Thankfully, I wasn't getting myself ready on my own – I had a team to help me, so I would look my best when I stepped out in front of the cameras. My hair was being blow-dried and styled, my make-up carefully applied. The make-up artist then began rubbing oil into my hands and arms and, as I looked down, I noticed something. 'My hands have changed!' I thought. 'They're starting to show signs of ageing.'

Immediately, a memory came to me of being a small child and seeing my granny's hands, wrinkled and covered in age spots, and thinking, 'I *never* want my hands to look like that.' I felt a jolt of sadness go through me. 'When did this happen?', I thought. Then I smiled at the idea that a young person would probably look me at me and say, 'Of course your hands look old, you're in your 40s!' What was happening to my body was a completely natural process so it didn't upset me or detract from such an amazing day. Nothing could – I never dreamed that I would be at the BAFTAs and I wanted to make the most of every second – but this fleeting moment did get me thinking.

One of my hands was burned in the attack because it acted as a shield and so saved my eyesight. As the liquid came towards me, before I even had time to register what was going on, my brain had sent a signal to my hands to protect my face. If it hadn't, I'd be completely blind.

When I spent time with other burns survivors during spells receiving treatment in France, I saw that many of them had lost their fingertips. It's a common burns injury because, as in my case, instinct makes you use your hands to try to put out the fire on your body. Doing this can save your life but so many lose more than only the tips of their fingers, they lose them right down to their knuckles.

I watched them learning new ways to do everyday tasks, like put on a bra or open a bottle. I was amazed by and in awe of their determination to overcome the additional challenges they faced as a result of the injuries to their hands. Knowing the impacts they would have on so much of day-to-day living, I thanked God that I still had my fingers. This is why I could never be so ungrateful as to hate my hands, no matter how many wrinkles or age spots appeared. Those hands had defended me and they've gone on to be strong enough to do thousands of tasks every day since – from grabbing my all-important morning coffee to holding the people I love.

It's so easy to take our body for granted – after all, it's always been there. But it is incredible. We moan when we have a runny nose, but that is our body flushing an infection out of our system so it doesn't do us further harm. There are creams to minimise stretch marks as they're viewed as ugly, but they are evidence of the fact that our skin can stretch and retract enough to accommodate a baby, which is absolutely astounding. We berate our brain for being slow when we can't remember someone's name, but it is processing an estimated 11 million pieces of information every single second.[1] Maybe we don't need to change our body. Maybe we need to change our perspective.

We have so much to be grateful for, but it's so easy to focus on the negatives, especially as we get older. It's understandable because prehistoric humans needed to be on the lookout for every threat that might cause them harm and, potentially, kill them. Life looks quite different today, but this human instinct has remained. We are literally programmed to look out for the bad. Social media throws further fuel on the fire, showing us all the amazing lives other people are living (or at least the highlights they want us to know about), and we feel we're missing out. Plus, all kinds of industries make billions out of us always wanting more and always feeling like we need something else to enrich our lives. Ageism, too, has taught us to focus on the bad things about getting older and look at what we may lose rather than what we may gain. We've seen the lazy stereotypes of grumpy old people who do little more than sleep in an armchair or hobble about hunched over with a walking stick. Most of the grandparents I know can still get down on the floor to play with their grandkids. They don't spend all their time moaning about aches and pains.

So how do we combat this skewing towards negativity that can sometimes feel like poison in our systems? For me, gratitude – being thankful for all the good things we have – is the best antidote. It can sound fluffy or twee, but practising gratitude has been shown to have huge, tangible benefits for us physically and emotionally. It can increase happiness, decrease depression, and improve relationships.[2] People often recommend identifying and writing down three good things from your day. One study involving adults who were seeking counselling services at a university found that those in the group who did this 'were significantly happier and less depressed, even six months after the study ended'.[3] It doesn't just make us happier in the moment, the benefits keep going!

I think that the more we focus on the good stuff, the more we see good stuff around us. It's like a muscle and the more we use it, the stronger it becomes. Think of it like you're walking through a field of tall grass. The first time you go, the grass gets in your way and it can feel like hard work. But if you walk that same path every day, it will get easier and easier until you'll barely have to think about which route to take in the future. The easier gratitude becomes, the more likely we are to be able to maintain our positivity on the hard days, realising that we still have the people we love, a roof over our heads, food in our stomachs, access to health care, and so much more.

Research has also shown that gratitude has physical benefits, too, including having fewer headaches, digestion issues and respiratory infections, runny noses, dizziness, and sleep problems.[4] We invest so much time and money in looking after our physical health, but this is a quick and free way to give ourselves a boost!

Gratitude doesn't mean that we pretend the hard stuff isn't happening or try to cover it up with fake joy. We don't have to act like everything is brilliant when it's not, but I've learned that there can be things to feel grateful for even then. If I make a mistake, I try to take what learning I can from it and be glad that I'll know better next time. If someone continually hurts me and lets me down, I realise that I can be grateful they've shown me who they are so I can decide whether I want that relationship in my life. When life is tough, I know that I will be more resilient when I come out the other side.

Sometimes almost losing things enables us to realise how grateful we truly are. I'm so grateful to be alive because I almost died. I have problems with my eyesight, but you'd better believe that I'm grateful that I can still see. Like all of us, I've seen people die too young and it reminds me not to waste the life I've been given. It brings into sharp relief that our time in this world is limited so we should make the most of it.

As I said, seeing other burns survivors who lost their fingers made me so thankful for mine, yet I recognise that I can still be hard on my body. We so often judge and critique our body using society's superficial and impossible standards of beauty that we tend not to think about what it can do and marvel at that instead. What if we learned to judge it neutrally on appearance because that is not its primary function?

We don't have to look in the mirror each day and rejoice when we can see more lines; we don't have to love every wrinkle and mark on our skin. Maybe some days it's possible and we can be happy that the crinkles around our eyes are the evidence of many years of laughter. But, let's be honest, sometimes it's not and that's OK. I have always been careful when talking about 'body positivity' as, having become disfigured at a young age, there have been plenty of days when there was no way I could have looked in the mirror and said, 'I am beautiful'.

When the trend for body positivity started on social media, it seemed really healthy for many – moving away from unrealistic ideal body shapes and, instead, embracing the fact that they come in different shapes and sizes, and all are worthy of love and care. But this, too, could feel like a pressure and unrealistic – that we have to be happy about every aspect of our body.

Jessi Kneeland, author of *Body Neutral: A revolutionary guide to overcoming body image issues*, says, 'We need to let go of the idea of body positivity. There's nothing wrong with loving ourselves or our bodies, if we're being realistic about what "love" means. But I do take issue with the notion that we should be able to feel a constant flow of celebratory happiness and affectionate gratitude toward our bodies, or that we have to joyfully embrace every dimple, every jiggle, every inch. That's neither realistic nor necessary. Body neutrality, on the other hand, takes the pressure way off, and tends to feel like a much more approachable and achievable goal.'[5]

I find this much more helpful. Instead of aiming for body positivity regarding the way I look, I now aim for body neutrality. I don't strive to love every flaw, I try to feel neutral about it and to place less importance generally on what I look like. I don't say, 'I love that I look this way', but I don't hate myself for how I look either. There are good days and bad days, as there are for everyone, but I want to be able to say, 'I'm just me and that's OK.' How I look is just one aspect of who I am and it's not the most important thing by any means.

I want to respect my body and rejoice in what she can do, and I know that's something I need to hold on to as I get older. I want to be able to observe the changes in my body without thinking they define me. Wrinkles are a change, but they aren't necessarily a good one or a bad one, they are just a change. They're not something to be ashamed of and hide but, equally, they're not a badge of honour that must be displayed.

As Kneeland puts it, 'Neutrality gives you space for everything that previously felt like a huge problem to kind of just be... whatever.

We're so used to judging and critiquing our body using society's superficial and impossible standards of beauty that we rarely think about what it can do and marvel at that instead.

Body neutrality can help us to take our eyes off what we look like, remember that our body is just a vessel, and put our time and energy into things that matter far more.

Not good, but not bad. Not something to freak out about. Not even a problem to solve. Sort of an annoying thing maybe... but ultimately pretty meaningless. It gives you the ability to see yourself and the world clearly, which means you can take your emotional power back from the places that don't deserve it.'[6]

I love this. Feeling negatively about our body can drain us, as we constantly feel like we need to change, and that's yet another thing we need to think about doing in our already busy lives. If we can't change for whatever reason, we may feel unnecessary shame. Body positivity can feel like another standard to measure up to, another way we're expected to gloss over something that can be hard and pretend we're fine. Body neutrality can help us to take our eyes off what we look like, remember that our body is just a vessel, and put our time and energy into things that matter far more.

Ultimately, we need to show ourselves and our body kindness as we age. Our body is incredible. We are incredible. We've come this far, it's carried us through the good days and the bad days, and will continue to do so. It will change, as it has always done, because of hormones or our season of life, and what that means we can eat and how we can exercise. It will be subject to illness, accidents, and the ageing process. But we'll never get given another one; this is the only one we'll ever get. Treat yourself kindly. You are worthy of care, respect, and kindness. Always.

A moment to pause
•••

What three things are you grateful for today? What would it look like to show your body more respect and kindness?

q

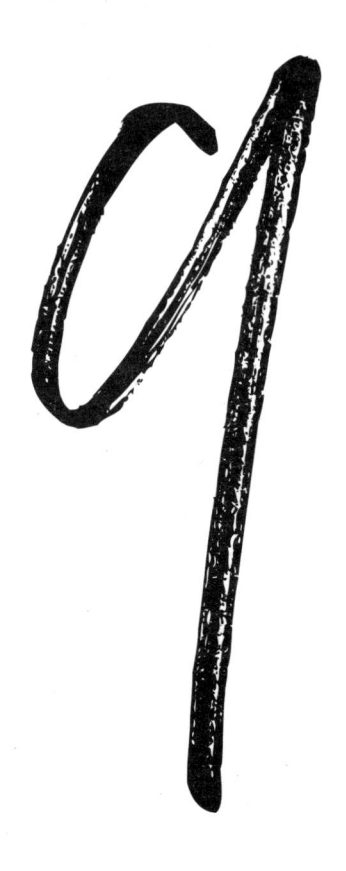

Take up the space

It seems to me that learning to take up more space is one of the best perks of getting older. What I mean by this is that, as we grow, we get more comfortable in our own skin, we learn to speak up, we are less apologetic about our needs and desires, and we grow in confidence. It's about becoming the most authentic versions of ourselves, finding the freedom to be who we are.

Sounds great, right? If you don't feel like you're fully there yet, neither am I. I can see how much I've grown and changed over the years, but I'm also looking forward to how much more of this there is to come in my life. Before we explore more about what it means to take up the space, let me start by telling you about a time I got the concept of taking up space really wrong and how it almost cost me my life.

Because I've had so many operations and medical appointments, I always dread getting ill. I've been fortunate that no one in my life has made me feel like a burden, no matter how much I've leaned on them at such times. My parents and Richie in particular have done a remarkable job of taking care of me when I've needed it. Yet I can still feel like I am a burden and don't like asking for help. I don't want to put anyone out at work either. I hate having to rearrange things or feel like I'm letting someone down if I have to break a commitment because of my health. I *want* to be dependable and reliable but, with my various health issues, there are times when that's not possible. This means that when I can plough on, I do – which, I think, is a common trait among women, and it's to our detriment. If someone is ill or in pain, we're usually the first to suggest they book a doctor's appointment or say they need a day in bed, but when that someone is us, we tend to just carry on, hoping the problem will go away.

I guess we've grown used to being in pain and discomfort since the first time we had a period. There are no allowances made for the fact that we bleed once a month, often heavily, frequently painfully, so we just get on with it and keep going, through school, work, and family life. And, all the while, we're told that we shouldn't mention it in front of men because they find it uncomfortable, so there's a tendency to keep how we are feeling to ourselves too.

When I woke up with lower abdominal pain a few years ago, I just assumed that it was the onset of my period and carried on as usual. It got worse and worse, but I didn't want to complain and have people think I was moaning so I stayed quiet about it.

I was working at an event as a keynote speaker, so I took painkillers at regular intervals and continued as normal. As the event went on, my vision began to blur and I started seeing spots. That might have been a red flag to anyone else but, because I have various eye problems caused by the acid attack, I reasoned that was causing it. My energy levels were dropping, too, so I felt exhausted, but I assumed this was because my life was full on and I was just overtired. I'm sure you can relate.

When I got home, I didn't stop and rest because I'd been away from my girls all day and wanted to spend time with them.

They were young at this point, with the littlest still feeding at night, so I didn't get a good night's sleep either. Nothing unusual there for a mum. The next day, I changed nappies and took my youngest to a children's play activity class before heading into work meetings, all the while feeling like I was in a deep fog, fantasising about being able to go to bed.

'I don't feel great', I said to Richie that evening as we stood in the kitchen. I started shaking, my teeth began to chatter and, though I felt freezing cold, sweat was dripping down my back. Minutes later, I started to shake uncontrollably and couldn't stand up. 'I think you're having a seizure', Richie said. 'I'm taking you to hospital.' He rushed me there and I was taken straight through to receive immediate medical attention after the nurses saw what a state I was in. They assumed the cause was an ectopic pregnancy because I was doubled over in pain but, when the results of my blood tests came back, they found that it was sepsis, so admitted me straight away. It didn't really make sense to me because I thought sepsis was something that was associated with a wound. I thought they must be talking about someone else.

I was in hospital for three weeks while they tried to get the infection under control. I lay there sweating, with my skin burning hot to the touch, but feeling icy cold. I was so weak, I couldn't even lift my fingers up off the bed. I was terrified by what was going on with my body and the grave looks on the doctors' faces.

After further tests, it was discovered that I'd had a simple urine infection but, because it hadn't been treated, it had spread to my kidneys and caused the sepsis. I felt so stupid. If I'd gone to see the doctor when I first started feeling unwell, this could have been resolved really easily. Instead, it became a life-threatening situation. What I know now is that, in the UK alone, there are 245,000 cases of sepsis each year, with 48,000 people losing their lives as a result.[1] It almost killed me – and all because I didn't want people to think I was moaning or let anyone down at home or at work.

Have you ever said, 'I can't be ill this week, I've got too much to do?', 'What if I go to the doctor and they say I'm wasting their time?', or, 'If I'm in bed, what will work/my family do without me?' Time and time again, we put ourselves last on the list of people to care about, treating ourselves in ways that we would never treat our loved ones. We pick up more and more responsibilities along the way as we get older, feeling like we're the ones who have to juggle everything, never dropping any balls, and inconveniencing ourselves rather than anyone else.

Why? Because the messages we've been bombarded with since we were little girls have been not to take up space. To shrink ourselves – physically and metaphorically. Diet culture encouraged us to literally take up less space, a physical reminder that we weren't to intrude. Most men have been taught to be physically strong, to bulk up their muscles, whereas the majority of women are taught to be skinny and slight. Men sit with their legs wide, spreading out as much as they please. Women have been taught to sit with their legs tightly together. We've been told in myriad ways not to be too big, too loud, too pushy, too ambitious, too human (basic bodily functions are not for ladies); to be good, be quiet, be selfless and unobtrusive. Speak softly, take small portions of food or be thought greedy, be subservient and don't challenge authority or risk being considered difficult. We were taught not to complain and rewarded when we smiled and made everyone else's lives just that little bit easier. No wonder so many of us grow up to be people pleasers – we were taught to put other people's needs before our own, to make them happy rather than make ourselves happy. We got used to reading a room, reading other people, and thinking, 'What do they want?' rather than looking inside ourselves and asking, 'What do I want?'

As recently as 2019 in the UK, supermarket chain Asda was blasted for the discrepancies between the messages its girls' and boys' clothing sent out.[2] Trousers for baby boys were described as suitable for your 'active little man' offering 'comfy styles that will mean he can be as busy as he likes'. However, leggings and jeans for baby girls were said to have been designed for 'a little princess' so she can look 'cute as a button'. Similarly, clothing company Boden had to issue an apology in the same year after the wording in its catalogue said boys needed clothes that could 'keep up' with their adventures, while girls were encouraged to fill their 'pockets (and wardrobe) with flowers'.[3] Another UK supermarket, Morrisons, was criticised a couple of years earlier for selling tops for boys with the wording 'Little man, big ideas', while for the equivalent girls' top, it was, 'Little girl, big smiles.'[4] All these things continue to reinforce the stereotypes about women's purpose in society: don't forget to look pretty and smile at the big, strong boys as they go off on their adventures. These examples aren't from decades ago – we're now supposed to be living in an age that's less sexist!

By the time we enter the world of work, we've picked up and internalised a lot of messages like these. The workplace was always a male-dominated space and, although we've come a long way, the shadows of the past continue to hang around. We're still not there with equal pay and, shockingly, only one in 25 CEOs of companies on the Financial Times Stock Exchange (FTSE) 350 index (the index of the largest companies listed on the London Stock Exchange) is a woman.[5] One in 25.

A result of this is that we can still feel like we should be as inconspicuous as possible in male-dominated spaces. We would never say that explicitly, of course, but have you ever noticed how the women around you apologise so many more times than the men do? I don't mean those times when someone's done something wrong and needs to make a heartfelt apology. I mean the everyday 'sorry' women say that just comes out without us thinking about it. 'Sorry if I didn't make myself clear' we say, even though we know the email we sent was crystal clear and the recipient simply chose not to read it properly. 'Sorry, but I just wanted to ask a question.' Why are we sorry for needing to have something clarified? We preface a suggestion with, 'It's probably a stupid idea, but I've been thinking…', putting ourselves down before we've even said what it is. Men don't tend to do this, usually offering their ideas without questioning how valid they are. 'I *might* be able to help you with that' is another phrase we use, even though we know full well that we have all the expertise needed for the situation concerned. When we need to ask someone to do something, we feel the need to add softening phrases like, 'If you've got time' or 'You'd be doing me a huge favour if you could' because when we just directed people to do things when we were little girls, we were called bossy, as though doing this was a bad thing. Boys are never called bossy; it's yet another derogatory term reserved for girls. We don't want to be seen as rude, conceited, impolite, or overly confident, so we apologise for every little thing.

Rae Jacobsen, in an article for the Child Mind Institute, suggests that a reason girls and women apologise so much could be because they 'are conditioned to be more attuned to – and responsible for – how their behavior affects others'.[6] Although girls are encouraged to be successful, they're also given conflicting messages to not be boastful, not upset others, and be polite, so they use apologies and qualifying language to downplay their accomplishments and ensure that they don't come across as demanding.

We carry these things from our childhood into the adult world, continually thinking more about how our words will land with the person we're talking to than whether we need to say them at all. When we do this, we can so easily take excessive responsibility for the impact our behaviour has on others.

The last thing I want to do is make anyone feel bad for doing these things. It's how we've been programmed and learned to adapt to what we face in the previously male-dominated world of work. What I do want is for us to recognise that we undermine ourselves when we act in this way, so it's not going to help. However, the modern take on how to get ahead at work can be toxic too – the idea that we need to act like men if we want to be taken seriously. Being like men is not the answer. Instead, we need to learn how to be ourselves in the room – the women we are when we know we are exactly where we're meant to be and we don't need to apologise for it. I love seeing older women who can do this, women who don't worry about how they're perceived and don't over-apologise. It inspires me that it is possible – we may just need to practise!

Part of the 'be a good girl' programming we inherited is wanting everyone to like us. This is not only nonsense but can also be thoroughly exhausting, as I found out. I was first known publicly as a victim and lots of people thought I was quite sweet. That's not a bad thing, but I began to feel like I always had to be over-the-top nice and worried that, if I didn't bend over backwards for people, they would think I wasn't really a good person and, worse, they'd tell other people I wasn't. It started to feel disingenuous, like I was playing a character who was sweetness and light and always had time to make everyone's day better. The reality, of course, is that I'm a normal human being who tries to be nice to people, but also has bad days and other demands on my time. Feeling like I had to put on a front and worrying what people thought about me all the time was draining. A light-bulb moment for me was realising that if everyone likes you, you'll probably end up not liking yourself. We can't be all things to all people, but we should be aiming to be someone *we* like.

Sometimes we have opinions that not everyone will agree with. Sometimes we have to make decisions that not everyone will be happy with. Sometimes we'll need to speak up and say, 'This isn't working for me' or 'I need this.' There's a risk that people won't like us when this happens, they'll judge us, think we're difficult, or divas (another word that has no male equivalent), but the alternative is to try to float through life, causing as a few ripples as possible. Is that really our goal? To have as little impact on the world as possible?

To me, to 'take up the space' means being unapologetic and voicing our opinions – something I think becomes easier as we get older. When we're young, we can have blind confidence in the idea that those who are speaking up know exactly what they're talking about, so we should be quiet and let them have the floor. As we get older, often we realise that's not the case, and we are now among the experts in the room. We've got experience, we've learned things, we've got a lot to contribute.

To 'take up the space' does not mean becoming an alpha male, changing our personality, or trampling over other people to get what we want. And it definitely doesn't mean pushing other women out of the way. There's enough space for all of us.

To me, to 'take up the space' means being unapologetic and voicing our opinions.

We've often been made to feel like we need to compete with one another, grabbing for the piece of the pie on offer to us. There's huge power in not playing that game but choosing to encourage one another instead, make space for one another, and help other women in whatever way we can. I love mentoring and encouraging women, whether it's through my charity, the work I do in prisons, or speaking engagements, when I get to encourage a room full of women to have confidence in themselves and keep going. Whenever women support women, I can feel the atmosphere change in a room.

Earlier on in my career, to take up the space in my workplace involved trying to convince people that I could do more than just talk about the attack. I had been blown away by the responses to my documentary and book and the interest people took in me, but I also wanted to move on. I was keen to work in TV, but the jobs I was offered all related to burns. While I was passionate about raising the profile of burns survivors through my charity, I also wanted to expand what I got involved in. With so little diversity among the people we saw on our TV screens at that point, many of those I spoke to seemed baffled at the idea of me doing regular presenting jobs that weren't connected with my injuries. It took a long time and a lot of persistence from me before people saw that there was so much more to me. I had to be tough and keep going, not be put off by the rejections. I started to say, 'What's not meant for me will pass me by', which helped me to learn to let things go. I realised that it was a waste of my energy to keep wishing that things were different. But I also had to be pragmatic. Some days, when it was all that was on offer, I would think, 'Maybe it's not the worst thing in the world to do another project about burns', but I knew that if I continued with that as my main focus, I would never break free. People find it easier to put us in boxes so then they know how to label us. I had to break out of the box and prove that I could do more than they could see at first.

One of the biggest things that can hold us back so we can't take up the space and live our fullest lives is the fear of rejection. If you fear that rejection will break you, I promise you, it won't. Don't let that fear decide your future – it can hold you back from work opportunities, pursuing your dreams, or meeting new people. I have been rejected countless times – personally and professionally – and I'm still here. There's almost a freedom to it (something many of us experience as we age), that once you've realised you can keep going after rejection, you try more new things, and then you know that the fear of rejection can't control you any more.

Writer and professor Roxanne Gay says that rejection of her work actually inspired her to do even better. She would give herself space to feel what she needed to feel, such as rage and sorrow, then would use any feedback she was given along with the rejection to improve her writing. She says that when women ask her how to succeed in the things they're passionate about, she tells them 'to take themselves seriously even if no one else will, to be undeterred in the face of rejection or setback, to know how to take constructive criticism and to know when not to take criticism… to be relentless'.[7]

I love this attitude and I've found, too, that being told 'no' doesn't always mean 'never', nor that I'm not good enough. It can mean that I need to adapt and change, or something might be for another time in my life. One person or company's rejection of us certainly doesn't define us. I love that Gay encourages us to take ourselves seriously too. It's great when other people see our talents and strengths, but we need to believe in and back ourselves, knowing that we have something worth bringing to the table.

Sometimes having confidence can be a 'fake it till you make it' scenario – you act confident and, in time, you'll become confident. Remember, you don't second guess other people in the room, so you don't need to second guess yourself. If everyone else *appears* to know exactly what they're talking about, chances are that half of them are just winging it and hoping they don't get caught out. Trust yourself, trust your experience, trust your gut. And trust that if you offer an idea that doesn't pan out, it's not the end of the world. We're all human and we're all learning every day – or at least we should be.

The world doesn't need you to have the same ideas as everyone else, to look like everyone else, to sound like everyone else. Being different is not only OK, it should be celebrated! I know what it's like to feel like you stand out when you don't want to. I can't hide my face and my story is out there for anyone who wants to know about it. As a society, we're getting better at diversity, but we've got a way to go. I still sometimes feel like I need to minimise my scars or health issues, try to find ways round the things that are physically harder for me, especially with my eyesight and, in many, ways it can feel like I'm trying to make myself more palatable. I'm far from the only one who feels like they have to tone down an element of themselves, whether it's their ethnic heritage, sexuality, disability, or just a part of their personality. In some ways, it's part of the human condition that we need to be able to adapt to different environments. We will act in different ways depending on whether we're talking to our manager or best friend. We'll come across differently when we're in the workplace than when we're in a coffee shop, and that's appropriate. Being able to read a room and act accordingly means we're socially aware. But there's a big difference between these situations and when we feel that we need to hide part of who we are, when we feel like we won't be acceptable if we show our true selves. To be fully alive, we need to be our most authentic selves. Brené Brown says, 'Authenticity is a collection of choices that we have to make every day. It's about the choice to show up and be real. The choice to be honest. The choice to let our true selves be seen... Authenticity is the daily practice of letting go of who we think we're supposed to be and embracing who we are.'[8]

The goal isn't for you to be like everyone else so you fit in. The goal is to be you.

We worry so much that if we show who we really are, people won't like us. At a physical level, I remember not wanting to go to the gym after I'd been attacked. I was still wearing the plastic face mask at that point and I couldn't bear walking into a gym looking like I did. I felt like a misfit and I didn't want people to stare at me, so I took up running instead. I had zero experience of it but thought that, if I ran on the main roads, at least I could hop on to a bus if I was exhausted. At first, I wouldn't make eye contact with anyone but, after a while, I noticed that the people I passed regularly started nodding at me as a hello, so I nodded back. This slowly progressed to saying, 'Morning!' and, eventually, there were several people who would have a chat as they kept pace beside me at different points on my route. It gave me such a boost in confidence and made me realise that I *could* join a gym if I wanted. It wasn't that I then knew no one cared how I looked because the truth is some people do judge; it was about me knowing that I would be OK even if they did judge me. The people who stare and talk about you tend to be the people who have low self-esteem. They do it because they're trying to make themselves feel better by putting someone else down. It's sad when you think about it – it's a miserable cycle for them and hard for everyone they judge without knowing their story. My bottom line is that I will no longer accept criticism from someone I wouldn't go to for advice. Our energy is valuable, so let's try not to waste it on worrying what people think about us when we can do so little to control that.

Guarding our energy and being authentic is an important part of self-care. When the idea of self-care for women first became a thing, it was all about having bubble baths, manicures, face masks, and spa days. Guess what? Someone else makes money out of that. I'm not against any of those things – they can be ways we relax and look after ourselves – but I think that true self-care goes far deeper than 20 minutes in the bath. Really looking after ourselves means being kind to ourselves so, for example, it's not only taking a break when we need to but also not letting the word 'lazy' enter our heads if we do. It's about taking risks but not criticising ourselves if they don't pan out in the way we had hoped. It's about understanding ourselves, owning how we feel, and being comfortable with our needs.

One of the women who has embodied this meaning of what it is to take up the space is Olympian gymnast Simone Biles. By 2021 at only 24, she was already being called the greatest gymnast of all time, with many awards to her name, including four Olympic gold medals. She was part of the US team at the Tokyo Olympics that year and the eyes of the world were on her to see what she would do next. The expectation was that she would win gold in at least three events but, after qualifying for the event finals, she withdrew. This was unheard of. Many athletes have stopped competing because of their physical health, but she was the most high-profile person to decide to do so to focus on her

I will no longer accept criticism from someone I wouldn't go to for advice.

mental health.[9] I know what would have been going through a lot of people's minds if they had been in that situation: 'I can't stop, the world is watching. People expect me to get another gold medal, so how can I quit? My team has poured so much into me, I can't let them down like this. Stopping would mean letting down my family and friends too. People will judge me for having poor mental health – they will think I'm weak.'

Stopping is not what 'good girls' are supposed to do. They are supposed to perform, to achieve, to do what they're told, and to put their needs last. So when we need to, we can second guess ourselves like crazy, with all sorts of lies running through our heads saying that what we're doing is wrong. Simone Biles standing against that and being true to herself is one of the most impressive things I've ever seen a young woman do. In withdrawing, she said that what she needed mattered. To every woman watching or who would hear about her in the future, she was saying loud and clear: how you feel matters, your mental health matters. More than any achievement. More than any standard the world sets for you. More than being a good girl and performing. You matter.

The world didn't crumble. People respected her and supported her and she opened up a conversation about the importance of mental health in a way that few could. As a gymnast, she came back stronger than ever for the 2024 Olympics, winning four medals. And when she was beaten to the gold medal for the first time that year, did she try to make the winner her rival? No! In a joy-filled moment, she bowed to her when she was given her medal.

If she could do all that with the eyes of the world on her, all the things she'd trained for hanging in the balance, we can learn from her – this woman who was so mature at such a young age

– and take up the space we need to. She did it when the stakes were incredibly high, so maybe we can do it in our everyday life.

I've also noticed that women in Hollywood are demonstrating what it is to take up the space like never before. When we were growing up, the women we watched on TV and in films would disappear from view once they reached 'a certain age'. Considered to be no longer sexy enough to play the love interest, the roles dried up, and they faded away, making room for the next doe-eyed young starlet with wrinkle-free skin to take her place on the conveyor belt. Not any more. Now, the women of Hollywood refuse to be sidelined. No disappearing quietly out the back door. They want to work, to be seen, to continue to tell stories about women at all ages and stages of life. Some have had cosmetic work done and others, like Pamela Anderson, are now so freed from society's expectations that they show up at red carpet events with no make-up. Of course, this doesn't always go down well or, at least, without comment. On reprising her role as Carrie from *Sex and the City* in the sequel series *And Just Like That...*, Sarah Jessica Parker said, 'There's so much misogynist chatter in response to us that would never. Happen. About. A. Man... Everyone has something to say. "She has too many wrinkles, she doesn't have enough wrinkles." It almost feels as if people don't want us to be perfectly okay with where we are, as if they almost enjoy us being pained by who we are today, whether we choose to age naturally and not look perfect, or whether you do something if that makes you feel better. I know what I look like. I have no choice. What am I going to do about it? Stop aging? Disappear?'[10] While she doesn't criticise other women for having cosmetic surgery, she's said that, for her, it's more important that she has full use of her facial expressions for her acting work than that she has a wrinkle-free face.[11] Her purpose in life is more than having smooth skin; she wants to show up as the actor she is.

Simone Biles and Sarah Jessica Parker are two completely different women being themselves and taking up their space. For us doing the same, what and how we do this will look different for each of us, at different times in our lives, and on different days. For some it will be doing big things, for others, it will be something small. It might be asking for a pay rise, saying no to something we don't want to do, telling someone we need help, applying for a training course, changing career, putting ourselves forward for a promotion, taking a mental health day, choosing what you want to watch on TV or which takeaway you'd prefer rather than saying, 'I don't mind, whatever you want', going to an art class, wearing bright clothes, having a sleep in the day, saying, 'That's not OK', asking for a second opinion, going to therapy, spending time or money on something that's for no one else's benefit but yours.

Sometimes the smallest things can feel like the hardest. When I have medicines that need to be stored in a fridge, I feel embarrassed asking if that's OK when I'm at an office or a friend's house. I don't want them to think I'm weird, but the really weird thing would be not asking! Like I said, I've got a way to go with this. We're working against a whole system of rules and ideas that we've been brought up with – a system that means other people benefit from us not asking for what we need and putting everyone else's needs before our own.

We can become so expert at pushing our needs down that we don't know what we want any more. I would encourage everyone to become more aware of what's going on inside and to start to take steps towards owning your life. Notice when you're letting your needs go unmet and ask yourself – kindly – why it's sometimes so hard to ask for what you want. Try to take up more of the space and see how it feels. It can be uncomfortable at first and other people might not always like it, but that doesn't mean it's wrong. You don't need to shrink yourself any more; you need to know your own worth. If you don't, who will?

These are lessons that it takes most of us our whole life to learn. We don't suddenly wake up one day and find we've worked it all out; we learn day by day, week by week, year by year. I feel grateful for how far I've come, and excited to see how things will look in another 10 or 20 years. I'm sure there will be different challenges along the way, times I might feel like I'm making really slow progress, but I want to remember that slow progress is better than no progress.

We've got to keep going, keep pushing against what we were taught about sitting back and looking pretty while men did the important things. Putting yourself last every single time could cost you dearly. Maybe because, like me, you don't take care of your medical needs, or because you spend your life as though it were someone else's. You are the only one who has your experiences, thoughts, feelings, ways of expressing yourself, desires, hopes, dreams. The only one who can live your life to the fullest is you, so enjoy your time on earth and make the most of it – you deserve no less. Be unapologetically you and act like you belong in the space, because you most certainly do.

A moment to pause
•••

What aspect of what we've covered in this chapter have you found hardest? Where do you think you already take up the space and where would you like to take up more?

10

Life is hard, but you are resilient

It was really tempting to write a book on ageing that says every single part of getting older is amazing. To lay out all the possible positives and gloss over the idea that there could be any negatives. But that's not life. It doesn't usually work out how we planned, so we can worry for hours, trying to be prepared for things that might go wrong, but it's often the thing that we wouldn't have thought of in a million years, the bolt out of the blue, that floors us.

The good news? You have got through every single bad day that has come your way. Every single one. There were probably times when you thought you couldn't take any more, but you're still here.

I found myself having one of those times not so long ago. I try to be a positive person and make the most of everything but, sometimes, situations are overwhelming and it's just too much. I had, again, ignored my health, thinking some problems I was having with my eye weren't serious and could wait until my next scheduled eye appointment. When I arrived for that appointment, the ophthalmologist was very concerned. He said that I had a detached retina, which had likely been detached for weeks. The injury, and the delay in treating it, could, he said permanently affect my eyesight. I was devastated, but there was no time to process anything as he referred me to a surgeon who was a retina specialist and I was taken in straight away for emergency surgery. I later developed some complications at home, so had to go back in to hospital, this time to a large one in London.

You'd think I'd be used to being in hospital, but I still find it overwhelming, especially one where I don't know any of the doctors. I felt incredibly vulnerable and it was particularly hard because my vision was affected and at risk. As I couldn't look at a screen or use my phone, I also felt cut off from my life. It triggered some of the trauma I went through after the acid attack, which heightened the stress I was experiencing. As you'll know if you've been through anything similar, it can be easy to catastrophise in these kinds of situations. I was petrified that I wouldn't be able to see again and what that would mean for me and how I would look after myself and the kids. I was worried that I wouldn't be able to finish all the projects I'd started and was passionate about, fearful of letting people down, and how we'd cope if I wasn't earning. Richie tried his best to calm me down, but I couldn't stop my mind from going to some dark places.

One thing about being in a hospital is that it reminds you suffering is universal. No one can escape it. It doesn't matter how old or young you are, male or female, rich or poor, everyone will know some kind of suffering. You might be the one in the hospital bed, feeling vulnerable in your thin gown, or the one who's at the bedside of a loved one, feeling helpless because you can't change things for them. We can think we're doing something wrong when life is hard, but things happen to all of us – illness, mental health problems, poverty, marital breakdown, miscarriage, cancer, divorce, redundancy. And we don't get to pick, just like we can't choose to have the perfect relationship, perfect kids, perfect job. Life can feel like a giant lucky dip and sometimes you win, sometimes you lose.

None of us can escape – bad things *will* happen. Perhaps, strangely, acknowledging this can help. It can feel like we're being negative but, as someone once said, what screws us up most in life is the picture of how we think it's *supposed* to be. We can get all sorts of ideas about how life will work out – relationships, career, health, wealth – but the reality very rarely matches up. Christmas is the epitome of this. There's so much pressure and our expectations are set so high that this one day could never actually be all we long and hope it will be, so invariably someone is upset or disappointed. Any other time of year, we'd think it was a perfectly lovely day, but because it's carrying the weight of our expectations of perfection, it will always fall short. The Christmas films don't help (much as we all love them) because, however nice your Christmas is, it's never going to match up to the magic of Hollywood, so you can feel like you're missing out.

Life is not a film, it doesn't follow a script, but even in films bad things happen. We'd find it pretty boring watching a group of happy people continuing to be happy and having no problems for two hours! What we tend to enjoy in films, is seeing people overcome adversity. Something in us recognises the story, even when our lives have very different circumstances, as we understand that this is how life works. We know that hard things happen and you work to survive them, change them, or make something good from them.

We human beings are hard-wired to survive. It's one of our most basic instincts, but we often say things like, 'I couldn't cope if *insert your own worst fear*.' Author Regina Brett wrote, 'If we all threw our problems in a pile and saw everyone else's, we'd grab ours back.'[1] Because we know how to cope with our problems, we're doing it every day. We fear the unknown, which is a good survival instinct, but it can mean we don't give ourselves enough credit for what we *can* handle. If we'd been told about the Covid pandemic years ago, how many of us would have thought we couldn't have coped, yet – hard as it was – here we are.

Someone once said to me, 'I would kill myself if what happened to you happened to me.' They weren't trying to be offensive, but this response highlights to me how we underestimate our ability to survive. I wouldn't have imagined I could rebuild my life either, but I have. The truth is, life can be hard, but we keep going. Having been through what I have, I know there's nothing life can throw at me that I can't endure. My confidence comes not from thinking life will always be easy but from my understanding of my own resilience. As a child, I didn't have a clue what I was capable of. Now, I can look back over the first four decades of my life and see a mountain of evidence that I can keep going no matter what. Whatever happens to me, I will rebuild, reinvent, and evolve – and knowing that gives me a quiet confidence in myself.

But it doesn't mean that I now sail through life without any worries. When I was in hospital again because of an infection following complications resulting from my detached retina, I was really low. So when we talk about resilience, I think it's really important for us to acknowledge that. People sometimes joke that I must be invincible after all I've been through and think nothing gets me down but, of course, that's not true. I'm just like anyone else who's been through an awful time. You fall to pieces before you can pick yourself up and put yourself back together again.

It's a common belief that there are certain people who are 'strong' and they don't feel sad or scared. As someone who has been labelled strong, I can tell you that this is not true. We are

You don't have to be a warrior every day, you can be a mess — it's all part of the process.

not machines, so we all feel things. It's part of being human so we don't need to put ourselves down for having such feelings or think that we're weak if we do. You don't have to be a warrior every day, you can be a mess – it's all part of the process. I think of it as allowing pain to visit but not overstay. We need to find places and ways to express our fears, disappointments, and griefs so they don't settle in and become part of us. Some of us may find we can do this by talking things over with a parent, friend, or partner; others by seeing a therapist or joining a support group; and writing down how we're feeling in a journal is also a good option. Writer and artist Ehime Ora explains what this does for us beautifully in her book *Ancestors Said*, 'You gotta resurrect the deep pain within you and give it a place to live that's not within your body. Let it live in art. Let it live in writing. Let it live in music. Let it be devoured by building brighter connections. Your body is not a coffin for pain to be buried in. Put it somewhere else.'[2]

Holding on to our pain weighs us down. We might think we've buried it safely but we're likely to find that it pops up again at some point, usually in an inappropriate way and at an inconvenient time. From my experience, learning to let go of things contributes hugely to strengthening our resilience. Lots of people ask me about the related subject of revenge and, personally, I don't find it sweet, I find it salty. I think the best revenge, comes from letting go, moving on, and living the best life you can. Anger, pain, resentment, hate, jealousy, shame – these are all normal, natural emotions to have in different circumstances, but none of them will serve us well in the long term if we want to keep going in life.

I've certainly experienced anger in the past, to the point that, in the early days after the attack, I would smash things up in my bedroom and destroy old photos and letters. I used to drink to help me cope, but I became very aggressive when I was drunk, so I started seeing a therapist, which was a much more beneficial outlet for my emotions. Some experiences trigger anger in me still, such as medical setbacks. When this happens, I don't diminish my feelings but try to write them down, talk with my husband, or go for as long a run as I can fit into that day.

There are many things that can cause us to be angry and, as we get older, it can feel like we've accumulated different ones, like souvenirs, along the way. They might be anger at a person or system, our circumstances, or our inability to change certain things for ourselves or the people we love.

Society doesn't quite know what to do with female anger. It doesn't want us to acknowledge it because that wouldn't fit with the idea that we are 'good girls' playing by all the rules and making life easier for everyone else. But we've got a lot to be angry about! Like all human beings, each of us has faced our share of hardships, but there are also so many injustices that work specifically against women, so many ways sexism makes our lives unnecessarily harder.

Violence against women and girls is growing rather than reducing. The National Police Chiefs' Council reported in 2024 that an estimated two million women each year are victims of violence at the hands of men.[3] It called this increase in crimes such as stalking, harassment, sexual assault, and domestic violence a national emergency,[4] but the structures and systems we have in place to deal with them still don't seem to support the victims. Many women fear coming forward as they're not sure whether they will be believed or blamed and belittled. Those who do bravely report such crimes are often met with misogyny when their stories are reported. Take Gisèle Pelicot, who so courageously pushed for her husband's trial to take place in an open court after he drugged her for years and invited men to come and rape her while she was unconscious. The original headline for an article in *The Telegraph* covering the case was that in doing this she was taking 'public revenge', but this wording was speedily changed when the public, rightly, reacted, pointing out that she was seeking justice, not revenge.[5] She wasn't retaliating, she was a woman who had suffered horrific abuse and wanted all those responsible to face the consequences of their actions. Weekly, if not daily, we hear horrifying stories of women who have been raped, abused, and killed at the hands of men. If we're not angry, we're not paying attention.

But because society finds female anger uncomfortable, we're not taught how to deal with it, but trying to hide it can have some unintended and devastating consequences for our body. Jennifer Cox, in an interview about her book *Women Are Angry*, explains that 'Our anger doesn't present very often in its straightforward form. It's disguised psychologically as panic attacks or OCD, and very often physiologically through chronic pain or migraine or fatigue. It is *displaced* anger. Other emotions come in such as sadness, tearfulness, shame, numbness and guilt. They push the original rage out of the way and sit more easily in our minds and within the role that society has carved out for us.'[6]

I find it really interesting that when we feel angry, we can look for a more socially acceptable emotion to express it, which shows me we need to keep reminding ourselves that anger isn't wrong. It's just an emotion that's trying to tell us something isn't right but, by us acting like it's wrong and trying to pretend it's not happening, we can end up with all kinds of awful physical effects.

So how do we let it out without hurting anyone else? Dr Cox suggests screaming underwater, throwing ice cubes on a patio, or whacking a wet flannel against a sink because the fast movement gets the kinetic energy away from you and into something else. Some of her clients get their frustration out by using a wooden spoon to hit a pile of coats. The important thing is to find ways to let the emotion out without causing ourselves, anyone else, or anything, harm.[7]

She's not suggesting that doing these things is a magic cure for what we're angry about. It's more that getting some of the anger out allows us to centre ourselves and then we can see what else we need to do about the root cause of the anger.

Something that helped me to let go of some of the pain and anger I've felt about what happened to me was finding God while I was recovering from the attack. Faith enabled me to at least begin to make some sense of the suffering I had been through. It also taught me it's fine to have questions but, sometimes, we need to stop searching for answers that we'll never find in this life. In my faith, I found a peace I never expected to, and I knew I was going to be OK, even though I was experiencing the darkest of days. I could accept that I was where I was.

Of course none of it should have happened but it did. My options were to use my energy to rail against the injustice of it or focus it on rebuilding my life based on my new reality. To truly live, I needed to start afresh and make the best of it. My attackers could take my looks, my youth, and some of my senses, but they only touched the surface, what they could see. My soul, spirit, and mind were still mine, under my control, untouched by them and untouchable. It took me a while to learn this, but it was a powerful lesson.

If I'd clung on to my anger and pain – justified as this would have been – they would have held me back and dragged me down, as any extra emotional weight we carry is counterproductive to our developing resilience. Doubtless there are many things you've experienced so far in your life that have hurt you. It's one of the realities of ageing that we will have encountered some of the most agonising things life has to offer, and sometimes it can feel like there's not much time to recover from one painful situation before the next one comes along.

As we process anger, grief and the other emotions that arise from these events, we need to lean on others. We may need professional support to help us with our mental health. On our own we can bottle things up, but professionals can help us to deal with our emotions. If you can't afford it and you don't have free healthcare available, find out about support groups as they can really help. Invest in books written by reputable therapists or borrow them from your library. You are worth the time, energy, and money, that may be needed to enable you to heal.

For the really painful and traumatic things in life, there aren't any quick fixes but, just like physical illness, it's better to take the time and do it well. When I was recovering from the attack, I wasn't able to work for two years. It felt like an eternity but, in the grand scheme of my life as a whole, it was important that I did everything I could then to get well. Now, all these years later, I'm so glad I did. We sometimes have to surrender and let things be what they will be rather than spend time and energy wishing that they were something different. In my case, I put all my effort into my healing and the court process and let go of any wishes I may have had that my life was like those of many of my peers, who were getting engaged, married, or having babies. It can feel like we're missing out but, as I said, life doesn't follow a particular timeline. What happens, happens, so we'll find more peace if we can embrace what is going on rather than long for something else.

Another thing I've learned is that we shouldn't fear the dark times – they are essential. Suffering is part of life, part of the human condition, and it's not all bad. We don't have to be thankful for every negative thing that happens, but we can often find there are positives that come out of even the worst events in life. I have friends who were devastated when their marriage broke down, but now they are much happier than they ever were before. Being turned down for a job we desperately want can be really painful, but sometimes a better opportunity comes along afterwards that otherwise we would have missed out on. During the Covid pandemic, so many people re-evaluated their lives and made changes they hadn't had the time or headspace to do before. Suffering can become the catalyst for change in our lives. It's a cliché but growth happens when we are at our most uncomfortable, and it often shows us the strengths we didn't know we had.

With the surgery I needed for my eye that I mentioned earlier in this chapter, there were some positives that came out of it. Richie advocated for me, took care of all the logistics at home, and bought me toiletries and PJs because I hadn't been able to go home to pack anything to take to the hospital. He was so kind and attentive the whole time I was unwell and drove two hours each way to sit by my side, even when I was groggy and not the best company. Seeing him upset at how much pain I was in was very moving. It's so easy to take each other for granted when you've been in a relationship for a while, but going through something difficult can help reset things and remind you how much you love each other. My mum came and took care of the

Suffering can become the catalyst for change in our lives.

girls for us and stayed on even once I'd been discharged to look after us, doing all the practical things that made such a difference. She even went above and beyond, cleaning the dishwasher filter, the plugholes, and the washing machine seal – now that's love! Friends sent me kind messages or popped in to visit when I was well enough and it meant so much to me. Times of suffering can remind you how many good people you have in your life.

It took me a while to feel better, but a few weeks after leaving hospital, I was able to run again. One day I found myself crying as I was going along, which is unlike me, but I had such a moment of overwhelm that I was able to run. I had been in a hospital bed, then at home, recovering, but now I was free! Free! I was in awe of my body – how she'd recovered, what she was able to do. I was filled with gratitude that I was feeling so much more myself again – something I would have taken for granted before I was ill.

I have been humbled and amazed at how many women I have met over the years who have shown such remarkable resilience in the face of some of the hardest adversities. Working with women in prison has made me realise how many of them have had to overcome an enormous emount, simply to stay alive. You will recall from Chapter 5 that I was scared the first time I visited a prison as I didn't know what to expect. That I would be crying at the stories I heard and inspired by the women I met was the last thing I thought would happen. Women are so easily written off by society and, in my eyes, never more so than when they've committed a crime, but all the women I've met in prison have agonising stories. They've had everything stacked against them from the day they were born, whether it's that they've grown up in poverty, witnessed violence at home and in their community, or had parents who told them that they would amount to nothing. There's often been a lack of education and opportunities, a lack of hope. So many have ended up in prison because a partner has coerced them into engaging in illegal behaviour, framed them, or they have fought back against violence inflicted on them. The Prison Reform Trust states that, in the UK, 'Many women in prison have been victims of much more serious offences than those they are accused of committing. Over half the women in prison report having suffered domestic violence with 53% of women reporting having experienced emotional, physical or sexual abuse as a child.'[8]

Maryam, an ex-inmate I met in the USA, blew me away with her resilience and courage. Her father had died when she was young and she grew up in poverty with her mother and eight siblings. As an adult, she made her fortune in property, but her whole life changed when she and her partner, Elton Thomas, were pulled over by the police. They were arrested and Thomas was accused of armed robbery. The initial charges against Maryam were dropped, but she was later charged with obstruction of justice. Though she denied it, she was given a 25-year jail sentence.[9]

When I met Maryam, she said she was continually put into solitary confinement, estimating that she'd spent about eight of the ten years she served in there. While she was still in prison, she was told the devastating news that her eldest son had died in a motorbike accident. This made me wonder what happens, on a deeper level, to someone when you incarcerate them. Are they ever really free again?

In Maryam's case, in so many ways her life has been horrendous but, rather than be crushed by everything she's endured, she's found her purpose and is using her experiences to help many other women who have been incarcerated in their difficult circumstances, and starting a charity called SisterHearts. The aim is to help women who have been traumatised by the prison system to heal and reintegrate into society. The charity runs an incredible thrift shop that not only raises money for its work but also provides employment for ex-prisoners. Maryam lets them sleep above the shop because getting accommodation can be really difficult when you have a criminal record.

I found Maryam to be incredibly inspiring. I could see the sadness in her eyes about all that she had endured but, at the same time, she seems to have an unbreakable spirit. Maryam did not forget her fellow inmates once she was released and has since dedicated her life to helping them, refusing to turn her back on them.

Alone in my hotel room the night after I met Maryam, I cried thinking about her, the violence and abuse she had faced throughout her sentence, and the sisterhood she has now created for others. I was humbled by having been in her presence. I'm sure she wouldn't have chosen to go through all she has, but she rose up, realised her strength, and made the best out of it that she could.

Of course, if I had a choice I wouldn't have gone through what I've been through either. None of us would choose suffering but, as the saying goes, no one finds their strength on a mediocre day. We only discover the depths of our resilience and our ability to endure when we're faced with pain and suffering. That's when we realise there are reserves in us we could never have known were there. Building resilience takes time. Kids have meltdowns over the tiniest of things, in our teens we may have been crushed by the smallest of negative comments or hard situations, but now, because of all the things we've been through – we're much better equipped to cope with things that are a thousand times

We only discover the depths of our resilience and our ability to endure when we're faced with pain and suffering.

harder than that. The more we go through, the harder the things we have to endure and work our way past, the more we learn and grow and build our resilience.

I still have my moments when I think that I can't take any more, but then find that, somehow, I have. I'm not only still standing but I'm also actually doing OK. All these things have taught me there is nothing I could lose now that would completely derail me. I'm not saying there wouldn't be things that would devastate me, but I know from experience I am strong and resilient. The truth is, you are too. Don't minimise this superpower, given to you by all the years now behind you. Recognise this power, take hold of it, and know that it's in your arsenal as you look to the years you have to come.

We don't know what life has in store for us. We're no longer in our youth with the feeling of immortality that comes with it, so it's easy to fear menopause and the changes it brings. It's natural to be aware that, over time, we will lose people we love, which will be painful. It's hard not to worry about what aches, pains, illnesses, and ailments we might have to deal with in the coming years, but we don't know what good things will come our way either. There will be people we will love who we've not even met yet. There will be places we will visit that will become firm favourites, ones we'll go back to again and again. There will be days of celebrating all sorts of things – new jobs, relationships, milestones, babies, and more. And there will be quiet moments that could be so easy to miss, but will be filled with contentment and feeling at peace with ourselves and the world.

It's good to remember that rarely is life all good or all bad. The day I phoned my mum to tell her the happy news that I was pregnant was the day she told me she had cancer. Invariably, when something is going well at work, there's something tough at home or vice versa. So, as you look to the years ahead, take courage from all you've already been through that has taught you so much and strengthened you in ways you might not have realised. Know that there will be tough times because that's how life works, but you are stronger than you think and way more resilient than you give yourself credit for. Enjoy all the wonderful, silly, small moments in life – they help you to keep going when the bad times come. If you're in a hard season, know that it is just a season – things will change. They always do. You have an amazing ability to adapt, grow, and change with your circumstances, and if we can be malleable, then we can do anything. Trust that your innate survival instinct will get you through whatever is ahead, just as it has got you through everything in the past. Take it from me – you are a powerhouse and you've got this.

So, as you look to the years ahead, take courage from all you've already been through that has taught you so much and strengthened you in ways you might not have realised.

A moment to pause
•••

Look back over your life and think about some of the painful things you've been through. Reflect on where, unexpectedly, positive things have come out of those hard times. Give yourself some credit for the fact that you've made it through everything you've come up against.

Making peace with death

It might sound bleak to mention death but, when you're writing a book about ageing, it's an essential topic to cover. And I promise this won't be a depressing chapter so stay with me! The truth is that if you try bringing up the topic of death with almost anyone, they will immediately try to shut the conversation down. We don't want to talk about it, we don't want to think about it, yet it's the only thing in the whole world that we know will happen for each of us. Not talking about it doesn't stop it from being true, just like talking about it won't actually make it happen. So let's talk about it because it's the final barrier to embracing life and ageing, isn't it? Living in the light of the fact that our days on earth are finite.

Don't get me wrong, I love life and don't want to die, but I've made my peace with the fact that I will. Partly because, as I've mentioned, there have been four times in my life when I've been close to death. None of them was how any of us would choose to die, which for most of us, I think, would be when we've reached 'a ripe old age' and peacefully in our sleep or surrounded by loved ones. And this is one of the things that brings up a lot of anxiety about death: the uncertainty as to when and how we will die.

Palliative care doctor Kathryn Mannix wrote in her book *With the End in Mind*, 'By encountering death many thousands of times, I have come to a view that there is usually little to fear and much to prepare for. Sadly, I regularly meet patients and families who believe the opposite: that death is dreadful, and talking about it or preparing for it will be unbearably sad or frightening.'[1]

It seems, then, that we're worrying about the wrong thing. If I had died at 24, I would have been completely unprepared. I had put nothing in place in terms of a will – not that I had anything to leave anyone! That's probably not surprising given how young I was, but you may be surprised to know that less than half the adults in the UK[2] and USA[3] have a will. In China in 2017, it was estimated that only 1 per cent of adults had made arrangements for their inheritance.[4] If someone dies without a will, there are certain rules about who gets what. For example, in the UK, if you are separated from a spouse but not divorced, they can inherit.[5] If you are living with a partner but not married, they can't inherit.[6]

One of the things that can make the thought of death so hard to deal with is wondering how the people who love us most will cope. The kindest thing we can do for them in advance is to get our affairs in order by making a will and leaving as many instructions as we can about our wishes. The last thing someone needs when they are in the first throes of grief is to be worrying whether we wanted to be cremated or buried, an organ donor, or they should bin or cherish our old teenage diaries. People fall out over who should get what, loved ones don't know which of our belongings we wanted to be kept for posterity and which were just functional and can be donated without a second thought. We can leave a lot of mess and confusion behind us if we don't think about all this in advance. The clearer we make it, the kinder we are being. Having these kinds of conversations is hard because, again, no one wants to think about death. But what's harder is not knowing what to do if you're the one left behind when the worst happens.

A positive conversation starter for the subject of death has been that people like Deborah James, aka Bowelbabe (who I mentioned in Chapter 7) and Kris Hellenga, a founder of charity CoppaFeel!, have shared their stories of terminal illness. Kris was diagnosed with secondary breast cancer at the age of 23 and set up the charity with her twin sister to encourage women to check their breasts in the hope of getting diagnosed early and, therefore, having a better outcome.

The year before Kris died, she did something amazing: she held a living funeral, saying that she wanted to 'celebrate a life that I have truly loved, surrounded by people I loved'.[7] Dawn French was there in her *Vicar of Dibley* costume, friends and family gave speeches, there was an ABBA singalong and a gospel choir. Guests were even invited to write her a message on her coffin with felt-tip pens. Kris said it was the best day of her life and, 'I've never felt love like it. I've never felt joy like it. I've never felt such kinship with mortality. I've never felt so alive.'[8]

Isn't it interesting that facing death head on can make you feel so alive? Kris knew that she didn't have a huge amount of time left, but her imminent death didn't become something awkward that no one around her could speak of. It became an opportunity to celebrate who she was and the life she'd lived. Hers is an inspiring example of what it can mean to make peace with death to make the most of life.

So we need to keep the fact that we're going to die in mind. Not morbidly ruminate on it, but realise that life is short and the only thing we know for sure is that we are alive right now! An awareness of death – even if it's with the hope that it is still decades away from happening to us or those we love – can lead us to be more focused, think about how we want to spend our time, and who we want to be. It can help us to cherish the moments we have, not take time with parents, siblings, friends, kids, for granted. If we knew we were going to lose them tomorrow, we'd soak up every last moment, every last detail of who they are and how they make us feel.

That I nearly died makes me so very thankful to be alive, but it has also taught me to surrender my life to a higher power. I'm no longer scared of dying because I believe in God and that there's an afterlife. There's a bit in the Bible that describes heaven: 'He will wipe every tear from their eyes. There will be no more death or mourning or crying or pain, for the old order of things has passed away' (Revelation 21.4, NIV). That sounds pretty amazing to me. I love life, but the thought of no longer having to deal with pain and operations, nothing that would bring me to tears, no more violence or devastation in the world, all sounds pretty good.

I also believe that whatever I go through in life, God is with me and will help me to cope with it. I'm not saying that I know what it's like to live with a terminal disease – my brushes with death have been short-term traumas, so living with the knowledge that you will die imminently is something that I wouldn't presume to speak on with any authority. Of course, it's especially hard for those diagnosed with something terminal when they're young. In my case, I had no time to come to terms with what was happening and, therefore, no time to really process what I would lose if I died.

When I first encountered God in hospital, I was at my very lowest – physically and emotionally – and, straight away, I felt like a huge burden had been lifted from me. My faith was then a comfort for me later as I rebuilt my life, so I attended a church twice a week. Before this, I had a lot of negative, preconceived ideas about what churches and Christians were like which, thankfully, didn't turn out to be true. The people there were so kind to me, answering all my questions, always encouraging me, and writing me cards to let me know they were thinking of me and praying for me as I recovered. The doctors and nurses saved my life physically and God, and the Christians I met at church, saved me spiritually. I found a purpose in life, a reason for living, something steadfast in a world that felt like it had been turned on its head.

If you'd asked me before all this happened, I would have said that I had absolutely no interest in ever going to church, but there was no way I could ignore what happened to me. The warmth, light, and comfort I experienced in that hospital room when I felt so utterly hopeless that I wanted to end my life were so real to me, I never looked back. I'd been to psychics before but soon realised that they only wanted to fleece me, frightening me by saying there was darkness in me that only they could cleanse. At a cost, of course. In contrast, no one in church wanted anything from me. I kept waiting for it, expecting that, at some point, I would be asked for money or to do something to pay back the kindness I'd received, but they never did. They restored my trust in people at a time when it was at its lowest.

I'm now aware of God's presence in my life on a daily basis and I wish I'd known this earlier too. It took what happened to stop me in my tracks and get me to realise that there was more to life than chasing after my own pleasure. In moments of despair, I know that I always have someone to turn to, for reassurance and love. It's the ultimate comfort to me, knowing that I would still have God, even if I lost everything else.

An awareness of death can lead us to be more focused, think about how we want to spend our time, and who we want to be.

I also have a lot of friends of different faiths, including a some who are Muslim, and I respect and understand their beliefs. I've seen religion answer people's questions about who they are and why they're here in a way I've never seen anything else come close.

When I was starting up my charity and working in an office that I shared with many other businesses, I knew a lovely Hindu man there. I was a mess at this point, drinking too much because I was depressed and always struggling to get into work on time. With my eyesight the way it was, although I was allowed to drive, I had trouble parking in small spaces and the car park at work would always fill up early in the morning. Bizarrely, there was always one space available no matter what time I pulled in, and it was always a wide one, so I could park in it easily.

One morning, I was making small talk with the Hindu guy and he said, 'I hope you don't think I'm strange, but I have a message coming through for you from the other side.' I wasn't quite sure what he meant and was waiting for him to be like the tarot card readers I'd encountered and ask me for money. Instead, he said, 'I have a message from Dorothy.' I froze. Dorothy was my mum's mum and there was no way he could have known that. We'd never talked about it, I'd never talked to anyone at work about her, and there was nothing online that would have linked us. He said in a very kind voice, 'She wants you to get help with something, something that's always making you run late. And she says she can't keep holding the parking space for you.'

I have no clue how he knew that, but it meant such a lot to me and spurred me on to get the help I needed to sort my life out.

I don't write about my faith to convert anyone or to be divisive – everyone is on their own journey, going at their own pace, and I make no judgements about what anyone else chooses to believe. All I know is that, for me, having God in my life not only gives me a greater sense of peace in the here and now, but also gives me deep peace about what will happen when I die. It's no longer something that I can't bear to think or talk about. And it's not something that has to be depressing.

I've found it interesting to see the rise in the number of death doulas. They help people who are at the end of their life in a similar way to how birth doulas help mothers-to-be and new parents with the ushering in and care of a new life. Alua Arthur is a death doula, founder of Going with Grace, and author of *Briefly Perfectly Human*, and she says, 'Societally, we shun death and make it bad or wrong because it's painful and hard, but it deserves the same sanctity as birth.'[9]

When asked what has surprised her about her work, she said, 'It's not sad all the time. There's so much laughter. There's so much love at the end of life. There's so much *life* at the end of life. People are most themselves. You get the best of people and you get the worst of people as they are dying. It can be beautiful. To watch somebody complete a life in a way that honors them is stunning. There's plenty of pain, I don't wanna discount that. But it's not the *only* thing. There's plenty of joy, there's plenty of color, and there's plenty of life.'[10]

She describes her work with the dying as being life-affirming and bringing joy, saying that it's the best job in the world, and I love that.[11] It's not what most of us would expect, but it shows that death doesn't always have to be a miserable thing.

We can't avoid death. There's no lotion or potion, prayer or incantation that can stop us from dying eventually. The human body is made to die. It's not designed to live for ever. Our body will slowly wear out and wind down over time. That's not a design flaw or failure on our part – we could live the healthiest life possible and still couldn't hope to live much longer than a hundred years. I'm not even sure we'd want to. Doesn't the fact that our days are limited make them more precious? If we were going to live for ever, where would the impetus come from to actually do anything today? Why not just do it tomorrow, or next year, or in the next millennia? Facing up to our mortality is surely the thing that helps us to make the most of our lives, really put things in perspective.

I don't think the opposite idea in the saying 'live each day as though it were your last' is helpful either. If you knew today was your last day, you probably wouldn't put any washing on or renew your car insurance. Assuming that you did live to see tomorrow, you'd be really glad if, in fact, you had done those things. However, it is more helpful to see things through the lens of questions like, 'How will I feel about this at the end of my life? Will I be glad I spent my precious time this way? Are there any broken relationships that I'd regret not mending? Are there things I wished I'd said?'

If we do have time to reflect before we die, there will be many decisions that we won't be thinking about – we are likely to focus on the big ones instead. Most of us want to leave the world that little bit better, and I don't mean by doing something dramatic like curing cancer (though if you can be part of that, all power to you – we would all be grateful for your contribution). Mostly, we want to make the lives of the people we come into contact with better – family, friends, colleagues, neighbours – even in small, everyday ways, by being someone who really listens or making them laugh. Maybe *that's* what people mean by living each day as though it were your last – giving all you've got to everyday situations and conversations and trying to make them just that little bit better for you having been there.

Let's not wait for a near-death experience or a terminal illness to

Facing up to our mortality is surely the thing that helps us to make the most of our lives, really put things in perspective.

start living as though we're going to die. Isn't it crazy that it takes something so final to get us motivated when all the opportunities are here for us to do something now? We can, of course, make bucket lists and think about places we'd love to see or experiences we'd like to have but, more than that, I think it's about showing up in our lives, living them to the fullest. That means being authentic, being ourselves. No one else can do that. It's the best thing we can offer, to make the world a better place.

One of the things that motivates me to live the fullest life I can is thinking about all the people who helped rebuild me after the attack. There were so many hands that worked on sustaining me physically, so many tears shed by friends and family who loved me, so many prayers offered by people, that I would survive being in intensive care, so much money spent by the National Health Service to keep me alive. Can you imagine if, after all that, I didn't bother to live my life to the fullest? If I had hidden away, like I was so tempted to, because I didn't think the world would want to see my face? That would have been crazy! I embrace life because I know, deep down, that I am blessed to be alive and I'm thankful that I'm well enough to enjoy it. We get one shot and this is it.

So my encouragement to you is to be courageous and embrace your life and your mortality. Be brave enough to put plans in place for when you're gone and be bold enough to live as though you've only got one go on this rollercoaster life. You are here for a reason. There is only one of you on this planet – there's never been someone exactly like you before and there never will be again. I believe that you were created uniquely, put here for a purpose, and I urge you to embrace who you are and what you bring to this world. We only get one life, with its tapestry of highs and lows, good and bad seasons, so let's remember to treat every day like the precious and priceless gift that it is.

A moment to pause
•••

If you were to find out that your life was going to be more limited than you'd thought, what would you wish you'd done differently? What decisions would you like to make in light of that?

Epilogue

When I was younger I used to think that my power lay in being physically attractive. It wasn't that my parents had told me that, I'd picked it up from the adverts for beauty products, diet foods at the supermarket, and the beautiful women covered in sequins who hung off the shoulders of the male hosts on TV programmes. Look pretty, be slim, and make men look good seemed to be our reason for existing.

Youth was the second most powerful tool for a woman and I didn't question that either. Until my beauty and my youth were gone – taken from me by an act of violence. In the years since, I've come to realise that I had completely misunderstood power. It was never in those things, which are impermanent, but in me. It *was* me.

As I've been writing this book, I've been reflecting on the many ways the misogynism of people and society try to take power from us. If they make you feel like you're not beautiful enough or slim enough, you lose power.

> If they make you feel shame for the things that have happened to you, you lose power.

> If you believe that your value diminishes as you age, you lose power.

> If they convince you that your purpose is to do what suits them, you lose power.

If they make you feel like less of a person if you're not in a romantic relationship, you lose power.

If they make you believe that you're not a proper woman because you've never had children, you lose power.

If they convince you that you're not a good enough mum, you lose power.

If they keep you quiet and stop you from expressing your needs, you lose power.

If they keep you focused on where you don't measure up to unrealistic expectations of perfection, you lose power.

If they make you believe that you are weak, you lose power.

If you've ever felt powerless, it's not your fault. Society was built on the back of it, but it doesn't have to be that way.

True power comes from within. It comes from knowing your worth, finding your voice – your unique voice – and adding it to the world in the way only you can. From carving your own path through life without the weight of society's expectations on your shoulders. Shrugging off labels others would try to put on you and defining yourself. Lifting up other women and allowing them to lift you as you lean on one another. Power comes from letting go of unrealistic expectations and impossible standards and, instead, being the one who decides what you want your life to look like. It comes from understanding your values and your place in the world. Knowing that your worth only increases as you get older.

I lost the very currency we are told makes women powerful, yet I became more powerful than some of my most beautiful peers. I had to rewrite my own narrative and find a place for myself in a society, where I had never seen anyone who looked like me. I believed in myself and what I had to offer the world and I found that there was room for me at the table. I've been given two doctorates, an OBE, and many other awards and accolades. Not one of them was for being young or pretty.

Finding my power was an inside job. No one could hand it to me. Even the people who love me most in the world couldn't do the work for me. I had to realise that it was in me and then step into it. As author Anne Lamott said, 'there is almost nothing outside of you that will help in any kind of lasting way, unless you're waiting for an organ. You can't buy, achieve or date serenity and peace of mind.'[1]

It's interesting that Lamott mentions dating because I think the traditional view is that the best way for a woman to gain power is to marry a powerful man. We'll let go of that myth once and for all shall we? The fairy tales told us that men rescue the women but, from what I see in the world around me, it's usually women who do the rescuing. You can be the power you were taught to attract.

This one is up to us. If we keep seeking power elsewhere, it will come and go, but if we realise it's on the inside, we can know that we will always have it with us. No one else can truly know what's on the inside of you, so don't let other people define you. You, and you alone, decide who you are. Get to know yourself, be the version of you that you want to be, stretch your limits, and see what happens. Make life happen rather than letting it happen to you. As diarist and essayist Anais Nin said, 'Life shrinks or expands according to one's courage.'[2] So muster whatever courage you have – even if it feels like a tiny shred – and expand your life so it is what you want it to be!

Call out the backhanded compliments. When someone says, 'You look good for your age', say, 'I look good full stop.' Don't shy away from people knowing your age and don't deny your life by shaving years off it. With each trip around the sun you have racked up more experience and more wisdom, so own each and every year.

Don't be confused about what power looks like. In the 1980s, the epitome of female power was women who went to the office in 'power suits'. You'll probably remember them with their bright colours and huge shoulder pads. There was something to be said for them – women who wore them were taking up space and showing that they weren't going to hide away. But, of course, power doesn't rest in a suit. You can be just as powerful in your scruffiest tracksuit bottoms because the power is in you.

People might be tempted to overlook, underestimate, judge, or dismiss you because of your gender, age, or how you look. That's happened to me plenty of times. I don't let it define me or let it make me feel insecure – I use it as fuel to show myself what I'm capable of. I don't do it to show *them* what I'm capable of because that throws the power back to them. And, ultimately, the only opinion that really matters is my own. So many older women talk about the power that comes from realising you don't have to care what other people think. Carol Vorderman said, 'I live without apology. Beware the post-menopausal woman who doesn't give a damn!'[3] When we don't care what others think of us, we're at our most powerful.

Let's not waste our lives. You owe it to yourself. And if you're struggling to believe anyone cares, let me tell you that I care. If you ever see me out and about after you've read this book, I would love for you to stop me and tell me how you've been living your life with intent since you read this. I want to hear that you are owning your life, at every age and every life stage. I want to hear how you're letting go of old beliefs that no longer serve you and realising how amazing you are. The more of us who do it, the more we will empower the women around us to do it too, and those coming up behind us. That's my dream – for the next generation to look forward to getting older because they see us doing it with pride and joy, and they see that our power grows with age.

Acknowledgements

I would like to express my deepest gratitude to all those who have supported me throughout the writing of this book. Some people may not even know how they've touched my life and inspired the things I have written.

First and foremost, to my incredible family and friends – your unwavering love, encouragement, and belief in me have been a constant source of strength.

To my wonderful team at Fresh Partners and Plank PR – for your tireless work, passion, and dedication in helping bring this project to life. You are all essential to this process and I am so grateful for everything you do.

To everyone at DK – especially Elizabeth and Jasmin – it's been a joy collaborating with you on this book. Thank you for getting it and getting me! Thanks also to Liza, whose insight and guidance have been invaluable in shaping these pages, and Michelle and Elizabeth for their hard work.

To the countless individuals who have shared their stories with me and inspired me along the way – you have all left an imprint on my heart that will last for ever. Your courage, resilience, and willingness to share your journeys have made this book what it is.

To all of you reading this – I cannot thank you enough. I know many of you have followed my story from the start and connecting with you – through this book, on social media, and when we bump into one another in the street – means the world to me.

Finally, to any of you who have faced adversity and struggles, who have been made to feel less than because of the way you look – I want you to know that you are not alone. This book is for you – may it remind you that there is always hope, and strength can be found in the most unexpected places.

Notes

2. What am I worth?

1 There has since been a huge surge in acid attacks. In 2023, for example, there were nearly 2,000 such attacks in the UK.

2 Georgina Lawton, 'Vampire facials, under-eye filler, "prejuvenation": How did cosmetic tweakments get so extreme', *The Guardian*, 6 May 2024, available at: www.theguardian.com/commentisfree/article/2024/may/06/vampire-facials-under-eye-fillers-prejuvenation-tweakments-cosmetic-procedures-young-youth (accessed October 2024).

3 Alex Janin, 'People are getting "prejuvenation" Botox shots', *Wall Street Journal*, 15 May 2023, available at: www.wsj.com/articles/too-young-to-have-wrinkles-but-already-getting-botox-2933eae5 (accessed October 2024).

4 Chelsea Ritschel, 'Resurfaced video of Victoria Beckham being weighed on live TV shortly after giving birth sparks backlash', *Independent*, 1 July 2022, available at: www.independent.co.uk/lifestyle/victoria-beckham-weighed-chris-evans-video-b2113900.html (accessed October 2024).

5 Daniel Welsh, 'Victoria Beckham opens up about impact of horrific front page telling her she "needed" to lose weight', HuffPost, 29 May 2024, available at: https://sg.news.yahoo.com/victoria-beckham-opens-impact-horrific-081106139.html (accessed October 2024).

6   Sarah Aswell, '*Bridgerton* actor Nicola Coughlan had the perfect response to being called "brave"', Scary Mommy, 7 June 2024, available at: www.scarymommy.com/entertainment/bridgerton-nicola-coughlan-perfect-breasts (accessed October 2024).

7   Jameela Jamil, Instagram, 18 April 2024, available at: www.instagram.com/jameelajamil/p/C56SNRMxl0q/?hl=en&img_index=1 (accessed October 2024).

8   Maya Oppenheim, '*Daily Mail* accused of "appalling sexism" for comparing Theresa May and Nicola Sturgeon's legs on front page', *Independent*, 29 March 2017, available at: www.independent.co.uk/news/uk/home-news/daily-mail-front-page-legs-it-theresa-may-nicola-sturgeon-sexism-compare-sarah-uk-prime-minister-first-minister-a7653556.html (accessed October 2024).

9   '*Daily Mail* urges "legs-it" critics to "get a life"', BBC News, 28 March 2017, available at: www.bbc.co.uk/news/uk-39421279 (accessed October 2024).

10 Mary McNamara, 'Column: Read my tan suit – Kamala Harris won't be taking fashion notes from the media', *Los Angeles Times*, 20 August 2024, available at: www.latimes.com/entertainment-arts/story/2024-08-20/kamala-harris-tan-suit-fashion-choices (accessed October 2024).

11 Carrie Kerpen, 'The biggest disadvantage women face in business today, *Forbes*, 21 July 2016, available at: www.forbes.com/sites/carriekerpen/2016/07/21/the-biggest-disadvantage-women-face-in-business-today/#125d0867cd99 (accessed October 2024).

12 'Beauty & Personal Care – United Kingdom', Statista, 2024, available at: www.statista.com/outlook/cmo/beauty-personal-care/united-kingdom#:~:text=Beauty%20%26%20Personal%20Care%20%2D%20United%20Kingdom&text=The%20revenue%20in%20the%20Beauty,US%246.65bn%20in%202024 (accessed October 2024, dollars converted to pounds sterling at same time).

13 Lollie Hancock. 'Global personal care and beauty market to reach £1,178 billion by 2027', Professional Beauty, 10 November 2023, available at: https://professionalbeauty.co.uk/global-personal-care-and-beauty-market-to-reach-ps1178billion-by-2027# (accessed October 2024).

14 Vanessa Van Edwards, 'Beauty standards: See how body types change through history', Science of People, 13 November 2023, available at: www.scienceofpeople.com/beauty-standards (accessed October 2024).

15 Indy100 staff, 'What being beautiful means in 25 countries around the word', Indy100, 15 June 2024, available at: www.indy100.com/news/beauty-around-the-world-countries-2668532752 (accessed October 2024).

3. Saying goodbye to the old you

1 Susan David, *Emotional Agility: Get unstuck, embrace change and thrive in work and life* (London: Penguin, 2016), p. 11.

2 Ashton Applewhite, 'Let's end ageism', TED2017, April 2017, available at: www.ted.com/talks/ashton_applewhite_let_s_end_ageism?subtitle=en&trigger=0s (accessed October 2024). Ashton Applewhite, *This Chair Rocks: A manifesto against ageism* (New York: Celadon Books, 2019).

3   Ali Xavier, 'The big issue: Playing the numbers game', *Therapy Today*, BACP, July 2020, available at: www.bacp.co.uk/bacp-journals/therapy-today/2020/july-2020/playing-the-numbers-game/# (accessed October 2024).

4. Own your story

1   'Sex attack victims usually know attacker, says new study', BBC News, 1 March 2018, available at: www.bbc.co.uk/news/uk-scotland-43128350 (accessed October 2024).

2   Brené Brown, 'Own our history: Change the story', Brené Brown, 18 June 2015, available at: https://brenebrown.com/articles/2015/06/18/own-our-history-change-the-story (accessed October 2024).

5. Finding purpose

1   Dr Julie Smith, *Why Has Nobody Told Me This Before?* (London: Michael Joseph, 2022), p. 280.

2   Fjohnson17, 'Closing the gap: UK fathers doing 18% more childcare since pre-pandemic', Fatherhood Institute, 19 December 2022, available at: www.fatherhoodinstitute.org/post/closing-the-gap-uk-fathers-doing-18-more-childcare-since-pre-pandemic (accessed October 2024).

3   Victoria Allen, 'It's official! Study shows women do 70 minutes more housework each day than men', MailOnline, 10 March 2022, available at: www.dailymail.co.uk/news/article-10596575 /British-women-doing-70-minutes-household-chores-day-men.html (accessed October 2024).

4   Emine Saner, '"The woman's to-do list is relentless": How to achieve an equal split of household chores', *The Guardian*, 15 August 2022, available at: www.theguardian.com/money/2022/aug/15/how-to-achieve-an-equal-split-of-household-chores-kate-mangino (accessed October 2024).

6. Happily ever after?

1   Julia J. Hynek, 'What's with all the songs about love?', *Harvard Crimson*, 23 April 2024, available at: www.thecrimson.com/article/2024/4/23/why-is-there-so-much-love-in-music-thinkpiece/# (accessed October 2024).

2   John MacGhlionn, 'Taylor Swift is not a good role model', *Newsweek*, 2 July 2024, available at: www.newsweek.com/taylor-swift-not-good-role-model-opinion-1916799 (accessed October 2024).

3   In the mid-1970s, 77 per cent of women were married by the age of 25, 91 per cent by the time they were 30, reports Nick Stripe in his article 'Married by 30?: You're now in the minority' for National Statistical, the Office for National Statistics' blog (1 April 2019, available at: https://blog.ons.gov.uk/2019/04/01/married-by-30-youre-now-in-the-minority). In contrast, 31 is now the average age to first get married, according to article 'All you need is love (and a marriage certificate)' on the UK Parliament's website (n.d., available at: www.parliament.uk/business/publications/research/olympic-britain/housing-and-home-life/all-you-need-is-love-and-a-marriage-certificate/#). (Both articles accessed October 2024.)

4   Rose McGowan, *Brave* (London: HQ, 2018), p. 43.

5   Zara Abrams, 'The science of why friendships keep us healthy', *Monitor on Psychology*, American Psychological Association, June 2023, 54(4), p. 42,

available at: www.apa.org/monitor/2023/06/cover-story-science-friendship (accessed October 2024).

6   Maggie O'Neill, 'Jane Fonda's tip for making real friends as you get older makes so much sense', SELF, 18 January 2023, available at: www.self.com/story/jane-fonda-adult-friendship-tip (accessed October 2024).

7   In an article in *Entertainment Tonight*, quoted in O'Neill, 'Jane Fonda's tip for making real friends as you get older makes so much sense'.

8   Dr Marisa F. Franco, Instagram, 15 August 2024, available at: www.instagram.com/reel/C-sUOfVOC_I/?igsh=MXhhcjNsM2V4dmgxeQ== (accessed October 2024).

9   Cher Fan Club, '"Mom I am a rich man" original Cher clip', YouTube, 4 October 2019, available at: www.youtube.com/watch?v=dZsL5R_CR-k (accessed October 2024).

7. Old is not a dirty word

1   Demography team, 'National life tables – life expectancy in England and Wales: 2021 to 2023', Census 2021, Office for National Statistics (ONS), 23 October 2024, available at: www.ons.gov.ukpeoplepopulationandcommunity/birthsdeathsandmarriages/lifeexpectancies/bulletinsnationallifetablesunitedkingdom/2021to2023 (accessed October 2024).

2   Hannah Waddingham's @ageismisneverinstyle Instagram account, 2 August 2024, available at: wwwinstagramcomreel/CLJSxRo20P/?igsh=OXgwdHRlcHk3MHhk (accessed October 2024).

3   Glennon Doyle, 'On deep self-care. Not breaking trust with ourselves', Instagram, 18 May 2020, available at: www.instagram.com/glennondoyle/tv/CAVIK9-hVgD (accessed October 2024). Glennon Doyle, *Untamed: Stop pleasing, start living* (London: Vermillion, 2020).

4   The Week staff, 'MI5 told to recruit more middle-aged mums', *The Week*, 6 March 2015, available at: https://theweek.com/62832/mi5-told-to-recruit-more-middle-aged-mums (accessed October 2024).

5   The LadyGang, 'Sharon Stone feels hotter than ever at 60', YouTube, 29 November 2023, www.youtube.com/watch?v=VRl5oyL-3T4 (accessed October 2024).

6   Greg Hassall, 'Comedian Kathy Lette talks writing, ageing and why she's putting the "sex" into sexagenarian', ABC News, 22 May 2022, available at: www.abc.net.au/news/2022-05-23/author-kathy-lette-on-ageing-disgracefully/100631352 (accessed October 2024).

7   Royal Marsden Cancer Charity, 'Deborah James – how cancer changed my life', YouTube, 27 November 2018, available at: www.youtube.com/watch?v=9qPbwDqKZZs (accessed October 2024).

8. A change of perspective

1   David DiSalvo, 'Your brain sees even when you don't', *Forbes*, 22 June 2013, available at: www.forbes.com/sites/daviddisalvo/2013/06/22/your-brain-sees-even-when-you-dont/?sh=c3f7d15116a1 (accessed October 2024).

2   Christina Costa, 'How gratitude rewires your brain', TED, March 2021, available at: www.ted.com/talks/christina_costa_how_gratitude

rewires_your_brain?utm_campaign=tedspread&utmmedium=referral&utmsource=tedcomshare (accessed October 2024).

3   Misty Pratt, 'The science of gratitude', Mindful, 17 February 2022, available at: www.mindful.org/the-science-of-gratitude (accessed October 2024).

4   Pratt, 'The science of gratitude'.

5   Jessi Kneeland, 'Why body neutrality works better than body positivity', *TIME*, 12 May 2023, available at: https://time.com/6279423/body-positivity-vs-neutrality (accessed October 2024). Jessi Kneeland, *Body Neutral: A revolutionary guide to overcoming body image issues* (London: Piatkus, 2023).

6   Kneeland, 'Why body neutrality works better than body positivity'.

9. Take up the space

1   'What is sepsis', UK Sepsis Trust, n.d., available at: https://sepsistrust.org/about-sepsis (accessed October 2024).

2   Rebecca Flood, 'Pretty awful: Asda blasted over "sexist" kids' clothes with boys' slogans saying "active little man" while girls' are "oh so pretty"', *The Sun*, 10 April 2019, available at: www.thesun.co.uk/fabulous/8832256/asda-sexist-clothing-parents-children (accessed October 2024).

3   Sabrina Barr, 'Boden apologises after children's catalogue criticised for gender stereotyping', *Independent*, available at: www.independent.co.uk/life-style/fashion/boden-sexist-gender-

stereotyping-girls-boys-children-clothes-twitter-a8761926.html (accessed October 2024).

4   Jonathan Mitchell, 'Morrisons sparks backlash over "sexist" children's tops saying boys have "big ideas" and girls have "big smiles"', *The Standard*, available at: www.standard.co.uk/news/uk/morrisons-sparks-backlash-over-sexist-childrens-tops-saying-boys-have-big-ideas-and-girls-have-big-smiles-a3596941.html (accessed October 2024).

5   Sarah Taaffe-Maguire, 'Glacially slow progress on gender equality as 96% of CEOs of Britain's largest public companies are men', Sky News, 4 October 2022, available at: https://news.sky.com/story/glacially-slow-progress-on-gender-equality-as-96-of-ceos-of-britains-largest-public-companies-are-men-12711481 (accessed October 2024).

6   Rae Jacobson, 'Why girls apologize too much', Child Mind Institute, 12 January 2024, available at: https://childmind.org/article/why-girls-apologize-too-much (accessed October 2024).

7   *Stylist, Life Lessons from Remarkable Women: Tales of triumph, failure and learning to love yourself* (London: Penguin Life, 2018), pp. 86–7.

8   Brené Brown, *The Gifts of Imperfection* (Center City, MN: Hazelden Publishing, 2010), loc. 866 and 876.

9   'Simone Biles withdraws from women's all-round final', Olympic Games, 28 July 2021, available at: https://olympics.com/en/news/simone-biles-withdraws-from-women-s-all-around-final (accessed October 2024).

10 Naomi Fry, 'And just like that… Carrie's back!: Sarah Jessica Parker opens up about a grand return', *Vogue*, 7 November 2021, available at:

www.vogue.com/article/sarah-jessica-parker-cover-december-2021 (accessed October 2024).

11 Perdita Nouril, 'Sarah Jessica Parker on why she's got no time for society's obsession with ageing', *Women's Health*, 7 November 2023, available at: www.womenshealthmag.com/uk/beauty/skin/a45720939/sarah-jessica-parker-interview (accessed October 2024).

10. Life is hard, but you are resilient

1 Regina Brett, *God Never Blinks: 50 lessons for life's little detours* (New York: Grand Central Publishing, 2011), p. 183, available at: www.reginabrett.com/50-life-lessons (accessed October 2024).

2 Ehime Ora, *Ancestors Said: 365 meditations for a peaceful year* (London: Hay House, 2021), p. 10.

3 Vikram Dodd, 'Violence against women a "national emergency" in England and Wales, police say', *The Guardian*, 23 July 2024, available at: www.theguardian.com/society/article/2024/jul/23/violence-against-women-national-emergency-england-wales-police (accessed October 2024).

4 Dodd, 'Violence against women a "national emergency" in England and Wales, police say'.

5 Yvonne Roberts, 'Gisèle Pelicot is a one-woman challenge to the still too common myths about rape', *The Guardian*, 15 September 2024, available at: www.theguardian.com/commentisfree/2024/sep/15/gisele-pelicot-is-a-one-woman-challenge-to-the-still-too-common-myths-about (accessed October 2024).

6   Jennifer Cox, *Women Are Angry: Why your rage is hiding and how to let it out* (London: Lagom, 2024).

7   Gaby Hinsliff, 'All the rage: Women are furious – and repressing it can ruin our lives', *The Guardian*, 3 July 2024, available at: www.theguardian.com/lifeandstyle/article/2024/jul/03/all-the-rage-women-are-furious-and-repressing-it-can-ruin-our-lives (accessed October 2024).

8   'Women in prison', Prison Reform Trust, n.d., available at: https://prisonreformtrust.org.uk/project/women-the-criminal-justice-system (accessed October 2024).

9   Marie Simoneaux, 'Ex-inmate launches thrift store to help others', AP News, 27 April 2018, available at: https://apnews.com/general-news-045310dfff3a4fd5a2911e3a65823758# (accessed October 2024).

11. Making peace with death

1   Kathryn Mannix, *With the End in Mind: How to live and die well* (London: William Collins, 2022).

2   National Will Register, 'Two-fifths of UK adults not discussed instructions after death, new wills report finds', National Will Register, 19 April 2023, available at: www.nationalwillregister.co.uk/news/two-fifths-of-uk-adults-not-discussed-instructions-after-death-new-wills-report-finds (accessed October 2024).

3   'How many Americans have a will', Gallup, 23 June 2021, available at: https://news.gallup.com/poll/351500/how-many-americans-have-will.aspx (accessed October 2024).

4   Hannah Gardner, 'Chinese don't have wills – and now it's a big problem', USA TODAY, 2 January 2017, available at: https://eu.usatoday.com/story/news/world/2017/01/02/chinese-wills-savings-beijing/95750124/# (accessed October 2024).

5   'Who can inherit if there's no will', Citizens Advice, n.d., available at: www.citizensadvice.org.uk/family/death-and-wills/who-can-inherit-if-there-is-no-will-the-rules-of-intestacy (accessed October 2024).

6   'Making a will', Citizens Advice, n.d. available at: www.citizensadvice.org.uk/family/death-and-wills/wills/ (accessed October 2024).

7   Kris Helenga's account @howtoglitteraturd, Instagram, 14 June 2023, available at: www.instagram.com/p/Ctct1hGteHT/?hl=en (accessed October 2024).

8   Helenga's account @howtoglitteraturd

9   'Death doula Alua Arthur wants you to live your best life', Keys Soulcare, n.d., available at: www.keyssoulcare.com/en_GB/connection/death-doula-alua-arthur-wants-you-to-live-your-best-life.html# (accessed October 2024). Alua Arthur, *Briefly Perfectly Human: Making an authentic life by getting real about the end* (London: Rider, 2024).

10 'Death doula Alua Arthur wants you to live your best life', Keys Soulcare.

11 Elise Loehnen, 'Loving the End (Alua Arthur)', Pulling The Thread with Elise Loehnen, 2 May 2024, available at: https://podcasts.apple.com/gb/podcast/loving-the-end-alua-arthur/id1585015034?i=1000654259659 (accessed October 2024).

Epilogue

1. Ben Yeoh, 'Life lessons: Anne Lamott', ThenDoBetter, 18 September 2017, available at: www.thendobetter.com/arts/2017/9/18/life-lessons-anne-lamott (accessed October 2024).

2. Anais Nin, *The Diary of Anais Nin: Volume 3* (1939–1944), Gunther Stuhlmann ed. (Boston, MA: Houghton Mifflin, 2009), June 1941.

3. 'Carol Vorderman announced as the 2024 alternative MacTaggart speaker', Edinburgh TV Festival, 2024, available at: www.thetvfestival.com/news/carol-vorderman-2024 alternative-mactaggart (accessed October 2024).

Sign up for my weekly affirmations plus exclusive updates on upcoming events and news delivered straight to your inbox.

Author Biography

Katie Piper OBE is an icon of her generation. A prominent author, broadcaster, and internationally recognised motivational speaker, she has been changing the landscape in the world of beauty for over a decade. She was the first woman with visible differences to appear in TV and billboard adverts for brands such as La Roche Posay and L'Oreal. Her charity the Katie Piper Foundation achieved Katie's dream to provide the first rehabilitation centre in the UK for people with life-altering burns and scarring. She continues to inspire millions of people all over the world with her bestselling books, her TV shows including her ITV breakfast show, her shows for U&W filmed in the USA, her podcasts, and her inspirational speaking.